THE LOST BIBLE

OF

HERBAL REMEDIES

Unlock the Power of Plants for Better Health

Healing Your Body the Natural Way

Emily Everleaf

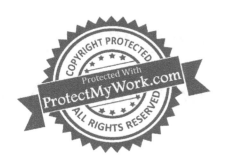

Table of Contents

Introduction

Welcome to a journey back to nature, where the power of plants offers a path to healing and well-being that has been revered through the ages. The Lost Bible of Herbal Remedies is more than just a guide; it's an invitation to reconnect with the wisdom of our ancestors, who understood the value of the natural world in maintaining health and curing ailments. This book is designed to demystify the world of herbal remedies, making it accessible and practical for everyday use, regardless of your prior knowledge or experience with herbal medicine.

With a focus on simplicity, this guide introduces you to the essentials of herbal healing, from understanding how herbs work to creating your own remedies at home. You'll find detailed profiles of medicinal plants, each with its own history, uses, and preparation methods, alongside easy-to-follow recipes that address a wide range of common health concerns. Whether you're looking to soothe a sore throat, boost your immune system, or find natural ways to manage stress, this book has you covered.

Safety is paramount when working with herbal remedies, and this guide emphasizes best practices to ensure you can explore the world of herbal medicine with confidence. From identifying plants accurately to understanding dosages and potential interactions, you'll learn how to use herbs safely and effectively.

As you embark on this journey, remember that you're joining a community of like-minded individuals who value natural, holistic approaches to health. The Lost Bible of Herbal Remedies is not just a resource but a companion, guiding you as you explore the healing power of plants and transform your approach to health and wellness. Welcome to the world of herbal remedies—your path to natural healing starts here.

Welcome to Herbal Healing

Embarking on the path of herbal healing opens up a world of natural remedies and wellness strategies that have stood the test of time. This journey is not just about treating symptoms but understanding and addressing the root causes of health issues. It's a practice that aligns closely with the rhythms of nature and the belief that the earth provides us with everything we need for our health and well-being.

For those new to this realm, herbal healing can seem like a vast and complex field, but it's grounded in the simple principle that plants possess powerful healing properties. These natural allies offer gentle yet effective solutions to a wide array of health concerns, from digestive disturbances and skin conditions to stress and immune system support. The key is learning how to harness these benefits in a way that's safe, effective, and harmonious with your body's needs.

As you begin to explore the world of herbal remedies, you'll discover how to identify, harvest, and prepare medicinal plants. You'll learn the art of creating your own herbal teas, tinctures, salves, and more, using ingredients that are often as close as your kitchen pantry or backyard garden. This hands-on approach not only deepens your connection to the natural world but also empowers you to take charge of your health in a proactive and informed way.

Safety is a cornerstone of herbal healing, and this guide places a strong emphasis on understanding proper dosages, potential herb-drug interactions, and the importance of sourcing high-quality, pure ingredients. With these foundations in place, you can confidently explore the healing power of plants and integrate herbal remedies into your daily life for enhanced health and vitality.

Remember, the journey to natural wellness is a personal one, and herbal healing offers a versatile and adaptable toolkit to support your unique health goals. Whether you're seeking to alleviate specific health issues or simply enhance your overall well-being, the world of herbal remedies welcomes you with open arms.

The Journey of Natural Remedies

The journey of natural remedies is a testament to the enduring relationship between humans and the plant kingdom. For millennia, cultures around the world have harnessed the power of herbs to heal and nourish the body, mind, and spirit. This ancient wisdom, passed down through generations, forms the bedrock of today's herbal medicine. As we delve into the realm of natural remedies, we uncover a world where each plant holds unique healing properties, capable of addressing a myriad of health concerns in a gentle yet effective manner.

Starting with the basics, understanding the properties of different herbs is crucial. Lavender, for instance, is renowned for its calming effects, making it a staple in remedies aimed at reducing stress and anxiety. Similarly, echinacea is widely used for its immune-boosting capabilities, especially during cold and flu season. This knowledge empowers us to select the right herbs for specific ailments, crafting remedies that resonate with our body's natural healing processes.

The process of preparing these remedies is both an art and a science. From the simple act of brewing a cup of peppermint tea to soothe an upset stomach, to the more complex preparation of salves and tinctures for topical application, each method extracts the therapeutic compounds of herbs in ways that maximize their efficacy. Embracing these practices not only connects us with the healing power of nature but also equips us with the tools to care for our health in a more holistic and personalized manner.

Safety, a paramount concern, underscores the importance of understanding proper dosages, potential interactions with medications, and the quality of herbs used. By adhering to these guidelines, we ensure that our journey with herbal remedies is both safe and beneficial.

As we explore the vast landscape of natural healing, we are reminded of the simplicity and potency of the earth's offerings. This journey is not just about treating ailments but about fostering a deeper connection with nature, leading to a more balanced and harmonious life. Through embracing the wisdom of herbal remedies, we embark on a path of wellness that honors the legacy of our ancestors while paving the way for a healthier future.

Importance of Herbal Medicine Today

In the modern era, the relevance of herbal medicine has surged, driven by a growing skepticism towards conventional medicine and a collective yearning to return to a more natural, sustainable form of healthcare. This resurgence is not merely a trend but a profound shift towards recognizing the intrinsic value of plants in promoting health and preventing disease. As individuals navigate the complexities of modern healthcare, the appeal of herbal medicine lies in its simplicity, accessibility, and the empowerment it offers individuals to take control of their own health.

Herbal medicine stands out for its minimal side effects, a stark contrast to the often harsh consequences associated with synthetic drugs. This gentleness makes it particularly appealing for long-term wellness strategies and for those seeking alternatives to pharmaceuticals that can strain the body's natural balance. Moreover, the holistic approach of herbal medicine, which considers the individual's overall well-being rather than just symptom management, aligns with contemporary desires for a more comprehensive approach to health.

Economic factors also play a significant role in the rising importance of herbal remedies. With healthcare costs soaring, many find that cultivating and using medicinal plants is a cost-effective way to maintain health and treat common ailments. This economic accessibility broadens the reach of herbal medicine, making it an invaluable resource for communities and individuals across various socioeconomic backgrounds.

Furthermore, the environmental impact of conventional medicine, from the production of pharmaceuticals to the disposal of chemical waste, has prompted a reevaluation of our healthcare choices. Herbal medicine, with its basis in natural, renewable resources, presents a more environmentally sustainable option, resonating with the growing global emphasis on ecological conservation.

The importance of herbal medicine today extends beyond individual health benefits, touching on economic, environmental, and social factors. It represents a return to basics, an embrace of the wisdom of the past, and a forward-looking approach to health and sustainability. As such, herbal medicine is not just a relic of the past but a vital component of a holistic, sustainable future in healthcare.

Part I: Foundations of Herbal Medicine

Embarking on the exploration of herbal medicine requires an understanding of its foundational principles. At the heart of herbal healing lies the belief that nature offers a bounty of plants capable of nurturing health and treating ailments. This section delves into the rich history and core concepts of herbal medicine, laying the groundwork for a deeper appreciation and practical application of this ancient art.

The origins of herbal medicine are as old as humanity itself, with evidence of medicinal plant use dating back thousands of years. Cultures around the globe have developed their own systems of herbal healing, drawing on local flora and traditional knowledge passed down through generations. This rich tapestry of herbal traditions underscores the universal human instinct to turn to nature for healing.

One of the first steps in understanding herbal medicine is recognizing the unique properties of plants. Just as each plant has a specific environment in which it thrives, so too does it possess distinct therapeutic qualities. Some herbs, such as chamomile and lavender, are celebrated for their calming effects, making them invaluable for addressing stress and anxiety. Others, like echinacea and elderberry, are known for their immune-boosting potential, offering support during cold and flu season.

The practice of herbal medicine is not just about knowing which plant to use for a particular condition; it's also about understanding how to prepare and administer herbs to maximize their healing properties. Techniques such as infusion, decoction, and tincture-making are essential tools in the herbalist's repertoire, each serving to extract and preserve the beneficial compounds found in plants. This knowledge empowers individuals to create their own remedies, tailoring them to meet specific health needs.

Safety is a cornerstone of effective herbal practice. While herbs offer a gentler alternative to synthetic medications, they are not without their risks. Interactions with pharmaceuticals, potential allergies, and the importance of accurate dosing are critical considerations. Learning to navigate these concerns is crucial for anyone looking to incorporate herbal remedies into their health regimen responsibly.

As we delve deeper into the foundations of herbal medicine, we uncover not only the practical aspects of herb use but also the philosophical underpinnings that have sustained this practice through the ages. Herbal medicine is more than a collection of remedies; it's a holistic approach to health that emphasizes balance, prevention, and the interconnectedness of body, mind, and environment.

Understanding the foundations of herbal medicine sets the stage for a journey of discovery and empowerment. Through this exploration, individuals gain not only the knowledge to address specific health concerns but also a profound respect for the natural world and its capacity to heal. This journey is both personal and universal, reflecting a shared human heritage that recognizes the value of plants as allies in the quest for health and well-being.

Building on the foundational knowledge of herbal medicine, it's essential to delve into the practical aspects of cultivating and sourcing herbs. This process is integral for anyone looking to harness the full potential of herbal remedies. Understanding where and how herbs grow, and the conditions they thrive in, can significantly impact the potency and effectiveness of the remedies created from them. Many herbs can be grown at home, in gardens, or even indoors in pots, providing a sustainable and accessible source of medicinal plants. This hands-on approach not only ensures the quality and purity of the herbs but also deepens the personal connection to the healing process.

Selecting the right herbs involves more than just recognizing their therapeutic properties; it requires knowledge of their growth cycles, harvest times, and preparation methods. For instance, the leaves of some plants may hold the most medicinal value when harvested in the early morning dew, whereas the roots of others might be most potent if collected in the autumn. Such nuances highlight the importance of timing and technique in herbal medicine, underscoring the need for a thoughtful and informed approach to plant collection.

Moreover, the ethical considerations of wildcrafting – the practice of harvesting plants from their natural, wild habitat – cannot be overstated. Sustainable harvesting practices ensure that these natural resources remain abundant for future generations. Learning to identify plants accurately is crucial to avoid depleting endangered species and to prevent the accidental use of toxic look-alikes. This respect for nature and its limits is a core principle of herbal medicine, reflecting a commitment to harmony and sustainability.

Preparation techniques also play a critical role in the potency of herbal remedies. Infusions and decoctions extract the healing properties of herbs through water, while tinctures use alcohol as a solvent, offering a longer shelf life and more concentrated dosage. Each method has its own benefits and applications, depending on the herb and the desired therapeutic effect. Mastery of these techniques allows for the customization of remedies to suit individual health needs, offering a versatile toolkit for natural healing.

The integration of herbal remedies into daily life marks the next step in embracing a holistic approach to health. Incorporating herbs into diet, skincare, and wellness routines can provide ongoing support for various aspects of health. From culinary herbs that enhance digestion to herbal baths that promote relaxation, the applications of herbal medicine are as diverse as they are beneficial. This everyday use of herbs empowers individuals to take proactive steps towards maintaining health and preventing illness, embodying the preventive ethos of herbal medicine.

Finally, the journey into herbal medicine is one of continuous learning and exploration. The vast world of plants offers endless opportunities for discovery, with each herb holding the potential to contribute to health and healing. Engaging with herbal communities, whether through workshops, online forums, or local groups, can provide valuable support and knowledge sharing. This collective wisdom enriches the individual's journey, fostering a sense of connection and shared purpose.

In embracing the foundations of herbal medicine, individuals embark on a transformative path that reconnects them with the natural world and its healing power. This journey is not just about treating ailments but about nurturing a deeper sense of wellness and harmony within oneself and with the environment. Herbal medicine, with its roots in ancient wisdom and its branches reaching into modern lives, offers a timeless and empowering approach to health that is both personal and universal.

History of Herbal Remedies

The tapestry of human health has always been interwoven with the natural world, with herbal remedies standing as a testament to our enduring relationship with plants. This bond, spanning millennia, highlights a universal truth across cultures: nature harbors profound healing powers. Tracing the lineage of herbal medicine reveals a fascinating journey from ancient civilizations to modern practices, illustrating how these natural remedies have evolved yet remained rooted in the wisdom of the past.

Ancient civilizations, including the Egyptians, Chinese, and Greeks, were among the first to document their use of medicinal plants. The Ebers Papyrus, an Egyptian document dating back to 1550 BCE, is one of the oldest surviving medical texts. It details a wealth of herbal knowledge, prescribing garlic for heart conditions and aloe vera for skin ailments. Similarly, in ancient China, the foundational text of Chinese medicine, the Shennong Bencao Jing, compiled in the third century BCE, categorizes hundreds of medicinal plants and their uses. These early compilations reflect a deep understanding of the natural world and its capacity to heal.

In Greece, the father of modern medicine, Hippocrates, espoused the healing power of nature, advocating for a holistic approach to health that included herbal remedies. His teachings, along with those of Dioscorides, who penned "De Materia Medica"—a five-volume encyclopedia detailing the medicinal properties of over 600 plants—laid the groundwork for herbal medicine in the Western world.

The Middle Ages saw the expansion of herbal knowledge through monastic gardens, where monks cultivated medicinal plants and translated Arabic texts into Latin, further enriching European herbal medicine. The Renaissance period further propelled herbal studies, with the printing press making herbal compendiums more accessible, spreading knowledge of plant-based remedies across continents.

Indigenous cultures around the globe have also played a crucial role in the history of herbal remedies, with a vast array of plants used in traditional healing practices. Native American, African, Australian Aboriginal, and many other indigenous peoples have long utilized local flora for health and healing, passing down their knowledge orally through generations. This rich diversity of herbal traditions underscores the universal human instinct to turn to nature for healing.

The 19th and early 20th centuries marked a shift towards synthetic pharmaceuticals, with many drugs being derived from the active ingredients found in plants. Despite this, the 21st century has witnessed a resurgence of interest in herbal remedies, fueled by a desire for natural, holistic health solutions and a growing body of scientific research validating the efficacy of many traditional plants. Today, herbal medicine bridges the gap between ancient wisdom and modern science, offering a complementary approach to health that respects the complexity of the human body and the healing power of nature. As we continue to explore the potential of plants to heal and nurture, the history of herbal remedies serves as a reminder of our deep-rooted connection to the natural world and the enduring power of nature's pharmacy.

Ancient Practices and Modern Applications

Bridging the gap between ancient practices and modern applications of herbal remedies reveals a fascinating convergence of tradition and science. Historically, herbal medicine has been rooted in the intuitive knowledge of nature's healing properties, passed down through generations and across cultures. Today, this ancestral wisdom is being validated and expanded upon through scientific research, offering a more comprehensive understanding of how plants can support health and wellness.

The modern application of ancient herbal practices is evident in the widespread use of botanicals in contemporary health and wellness industries. Adaptogens, a class of herbs known for their ability to help the body resist stressors, are a prime example of ancient remedies gaining prominence in today's health-conscious society. Herbs like ashwagandha, used for centuries in Ayurvedic medicine to bolster the immune system and combat stress, are now featured in supplements, teas, and wellness products globally. This fusion of ancient knowledge with modern consumption patterns underscores the timeless relevance of herbal remedies.

Incorporating herbal practices into modern healthcare also involves a renewed focus on holistic treatment approaches. Rather than isolating symptoms, herbal medicine encourages a comprehensive view of the individual's health, considering physical, emotional, and environmental factors. This holistic perspective, deeply rooted in traditional herbalism, is gaining traction in modern medicine as more healthcare practitioners recognize the limitations of a purely symptom-focused approach.

The resurgence of herbal gardens and community-supported agriculture (CSA) programs reflects a growing desire to reconnect with the source of our remedies. People are increasingly interested in growing their own medicinal plants, mirroring the ancient practice of cultivating personal herb gardens. This hands-on approach not only fosters a deeper connection with the healing process but also ensures access to fresh, potent botanicals. Modern applications extend to urban environments where community gardens and indoor herbal cultivation kits make herbal practices accessible to a wider audience.

Technological advancements have further transformed how we engage with herbal remedies. Digital platforms offer unprecedented access to herbal knowledge, from online courses on herbalism to apps that help identify medicinal plants in the wild. This democratization of knowledge empowers individuals to explore herbal remedies with confidence, guided by both ancient wisdom and contemporary science.

Moreover, the integration of herbal remedies into daily life has evolved with modern needs and lifestyles. Innovative product formulations and convenient delivery systems, such as herbal patches, capsules, and sprays, cater to the fast-paced lives of today's consumers while preserving the essence of traditional herbal practices. These developments signify a broader acceptance and integration of herbal medicine into mainstream health and wellness routines.

As we navigate the complexities of modern life, the principles of ancient herbal practices offer grounding and guidance. By embracing the synergy between tradition and innovation, we can harness the full potential of herbal remedies to support a holistic, balanced approach to health and well-being. The journey of herbal medicine, from ancient practices to modern applications, illustrates a collective aspiration to live in harmony with nature, drawing on its profound capacity to heal.

Cultural Significance of Herbs

Herbs have woven their way through the tapestry of human culture, marking significant impacts on culinary traditions, medicinal practices, and spiritual rituals across the globe. Their cultural significance is as diverse as the plants themselves, reflecting the unique relationships between different societies and the natural world. From the sacred basil (Tulsi) revered in Indian spirituality to the white sage used in Native American cleansing ceremonies, herbs carry profound meanings and uses that transcend their physical properties.

In many cultures, herbs are deeply entwined with traditional healing practices, serving as the foundation for age-old remedies passed down through generations. For instance, Chinese medicine, with its roots stretching back thousands of years, utilizes an extensive pharmacopeia of herbs in complex formulas designed to balance the body's Qi. Similarly, in Western herbalism, plants like lavender and chamomile have been used since the time of the ancient Greeks and Romans for their calming and healing effects, illustrating a long-standing appreciation for the soothing power of herbs.

The culinary use of herbs is another realm where their cultural significance shines. Herbs are not merely ingredients; they are carriers of flavor, tradition, and identity. The use of rosemary in Italian cooking, cilantro in Mexican cuisine, or mint in Middle Eastern dishes speaks volumes about the regional preferences and agricultural practices that shape local foodways. These culinary traditions, enriched by the use of herbs, offer a window into the cultural landscapes from which they emerge, highlighting the role of herbs in celebrating and preserving cultural heritage.

Spiritually, herbs occupy a sacred space in many religions and belief systems, used in rituals and ceremonies to purify, protect, and connect with the divine. The burning of frankincense in Christian churches, the use of sweetgrass in Indigenous smudging ceremonies, and the offering of marigolds in Hindu rituals exemplify the spiritual dimensions of herbs. These practices underscore the belief in the transcendent power of plants to bridge the earthly and the divine, facilitating communication with spiritual realms and enhancing the sacredness of ritual acts.

The cultural significance of herbs also extends to their symbolic meanings. In many societies, herbs symbolize love, protection, health, and prosperity. The giving of rosemary at weddings as a symbol of fidelity, the hanging of eucalyptus for protection, or the placing of basil in a pot by the front door to ensure prosperity are all practices imbued with symbolic meanings, reflecting the deep connections people have with these plants beyond their tangible benefits.

In contemporary times, the cultural significance of herbs is being rediscovered and embraced in new ways, as people seek to reconnect with the natural world and explore the wisdom of traditional herbal practices. This resurgence of interest in herbalism is not just a return to the past but a vibrant reimagining of how herbs can enrich our lives, promote wellness, and deepen our connection to our cultural roots and the earth.

As we continue to explore and appreciate the multifaceted roles of herbs in human culture, we are reminded of the enduring power of plants to nourish, heal, and inspire. The cultural significance of herbs, with its rich tapestry of meanings, uses, and traditions, offers a profound testament to the integral role these plants have played—and continue to play—in the human journey.

Understanding Herbal Medicine

Herbal medicine, often referred to as botanical medicine or phytotherapy, involves using plant-based materials for therapeutic purposes. This ancient practice, deeply rooted in the world's history, harnesses the healing power of plants to treat various ailments and promote overall well-being. It operates on the principle that plants contain natural substances that can enhance the body's health and healing capabilities.

At the core of herbal medicine is the belief that each plant has a unique profile of active compounds, known as phytochemicals, which can exert therapeutic effects on the human body. These compounds can work individually or synergistically to prevent, alleviate, or cure diseases. Understanding the properties and uses of these plants requires a blend of traditional knowledge and modern scientific research.

One fundamental aspect of herbal medicine is the holistic approach to treatment. Unlike conventional medicine, which often focuses on treating specific symptoms, herbal medicine looks at the individual's overall condition, seeking to address the root cause of health issues. This approach not only aims to treat the immediate problem but also to enhance the body's own healing mechanisms and support long-term health and vitality.

For beginners, it's essential to grasp the basics of how to safely and effectively use herbs. This includes learning about different forms of herbal preparations such as teas, tinctures, capsules, and topicals. Each preparation method extracts the active compounds in ways that are most suitable for treating specific conditions. For instance, teas may be beneficial for their soothing and hydrating properties, while tinctures offer a more concentrated form of the herb for more potent therapeutic effects.

Safety is a paramount concern in herbal medicine. While herbs are natural, they are not inherently without risk. Interactions with prescription medications, possible side effects, and individual allergies are critical considerations. Proper dosing is also crucial, as the therapeutic window—the range between effectiveness and toxicity—can vary widely among different herbs and individuals.

Quality and sourcing of herbs are other important factors. The potency and safety of herbal remedies can be influenced by where and how the plants are grown, harvested, and processed. Opting for organically grown herbs and reputable sources can help ensure the purity and efficacy of the remedies you use.

For those looking to integrate herbal medicine into their health regimen, starting with a few simple, well-researched herbs is advisable. Familiarizing oneself with these plants, their uses, and proper preparation methods can provide a solid foundation for further exploration into the vast world of herbal remedies.

Herbal medicine offers a rich and accessible way to enhance health and well-being, drawing on the synergy between nature and the human body. By combining ancient wisdom with modern science, individuals can unlock the healing power of plants and take an active role in their health journey. As with any healthcare approach, it's essential to proceed with knowledge, caution, and respect for the natural world's complexity and power.

How Herbal Remedies Work

Herbal remedies work by utilizing the natural compounds found in plants, known as phytochemicals, to promote healing and well-being within the body. These phytochemicals include a wide range of substances such as essential oils, flavonoids, alkaloids, and terpenoids, each with unique therapeutic properties. When consumed or applied, these compounds interact with the body's biological systems, triggering responses that can help to prevent, alleviate, or cure various health conditions.

The effectiveness of herbal remedies is rooted in their ability to work in harmony with the body's own healing mechanisms. Unlike many synthetic drugs that often target a specific area or symptom, herbs can provide a more holistic benefit. For example, some herbs may have anti-inflammatory properties that help reduce swelling and pain, while others may boost the immune system, helping the body to fight off infections more effectively.

One of the key ways herbal remedies exert their effects is through the modulation of the body's own biochemical pathways. For instance, certain herbs can influence the body's production of hormones and neurotransmitters, which play crucial roles in mood regulation, stress response, and overall mental health. Herbs like St. John's Wort, known for its antidepressant properties, work by affecting neurotransmitters such as serotonin and dopamine, thereby improving mood and alleviating symptoms of depression.

Herbal remedies also support detoxification and cleansing processes in the body. Many herbs enhance liver function, which is pivotal in the detoxification of harmful substances from the body. Dandelion root and milk thistle are well-known for their liver-supportive properties, helping to cleanse the body and improve overall health.

Digestive health is another area where herbal remedies shine. Many herbs stimulate digestion, reduce inflammation in the gastrointestinal tract, and alleviate symptoms of discomfort. Peppermint, for example, has been shown to relax the muscles of the digestive tract, easing symptoms of irritable bowel syndrome (IBS) and indigestion.

Safety in the use of herbal remedies is paramount, and understanding the correct dosages, potential interactions with medications, and the quality of herbs used is essential for achieving the desired therapeutic outcomes without adverse effects. It's also crucial to recognize that individual responses to herbal remedies can vary, and what works for one person may not work for another, underscoring the importance of personalized herbal medicine.

In summary, herbal remedies offer a natural, effective way to support health and well-being, working in conjunction with the body's own processes to heal and maintain balance. Through the careful selection and application of specific herbs, individuals can harness the power of nature to address a wide range of health concerns, from mental health issues to digestive disorders, in a holistic and integrative manner.

Science Behind Herbal Medicine

Herbal medicine harnesses the intricate chemistry of plants, tapping into a vast array of phytochemicals that have evolved over millennia. These natural compounds, such as alkaloids, flavonoids, and terpenes, interact with the human body in complex ways, often mirroring the actions of pharmaceuticals but with a key difference: they tend to work more synergistically with the body's own systems. The science behind herbal medicine is grounded in understanding these interactions and the physiological effects they elicit.

At the heart of herbal medicine is the principle of synergy, where the combined effect of a plant's compounds is greater than the sum of its individual components. This contrasts with conventional drugs, which typically isolate a single active ingredient. The holistic nature of herbal medicine means that multiple pathways in the body can be supported or modulated at once, contributing to its effectiveness in treating the whole person rather than just addressing symptoms.

Research into the science of herbal medicine often focuses on identifying active compounds and understanding their mechanisms of action. For instance, studies have shown that salicin, found in white willow bark, is converted by the body into salicylic acid, the basis for aspirin, providing pain relief and anti-inflammatory effects. Similarly, the sedative properties of valerian root are attributed to valepotriates and valerenic acid, which influence GABA receptors in the brain, helping to reduce anxiety and improve sleep quality.

Pharmacokinetics, or how the body absorbs, distributes, metabolizes, and excretes these compounds, is another crucial aspect. Many herbs act as adaptogens, helping to modulate the body's stress response by affecting hormone levels and physiological pathways. This adaptogenic action illustrates the body's remarkable ability to use plant compounds to restore balance and resilience to stress.

Safety and efficacy are paramount, and the science of herbal medicine includes rigorous testing and validation. Clinical trials, ethnobotanical studies, and pharmacological research contribute to our understanding of how best to use these natural remedies. While the complexity of plant matrices can pose challenges for standardization and quality control, advancements in analytical techniques are improving the reliability and consistency of herbal products.

Understanding the science behind herbal medicine empowers individuals to make informed choices about their health. It bridges traditional knowledge with modern scientific inquiry, validating the use of plants as medicine and offering a complementary approach to health care that is both ancient and profoundly relevant today. This knowledge equips us to navigate the vast world of herbal remedies with confidence, respecting both the power of nature and the body's innate healing capabilities.

Safety and Precautions

When embarking on the exploration of herbal remedies, prioritizing safety and precautions is essential to ensure that the journey towards natural healing remains beneficial and devoid of adverse effects. The allure of harnessing nature's bounty to support health and well-being is undeniable, yet it comes with the responsibility of understanding and respecting the potency and potential risks associated with medicinal plants. As beginners in the realm of herbal medicine, it is crucial to approach this practice with a mindset that values informed decision-making, meticulous research, and adherence to guidelines that safeguard health.

First and foremost, accurate identification of herbs is paramount. Misidentifying a plant can lead to the use of a potentially harmful species, negating the healing intentions and possibly causing adverse reactions. Therefore, consulting reliable sources, such as reputable herbal guides or professionals in botanical medicine, is a step that cannot be overlooked. When foraging for herbs in the wild, this becomes even more critical, as the risk of mistaking one plant for another increases.

Understanding dosages is another cornerstone of safe herbal practice. Just as with conventional medicines, the principle of "the dose makes the poison" applies. Consuming too much of an herb can lead to toxicity, while too little may render the remedy ineffective. Familiarizing oneself with the recommended dosages for specific conditions and starting with the lower end of the dosage spectrum can help mitigate risks. It is also advisable to keep a record of the herbs used, their dosages, and any reactions experienced, as this information can be invaluable for both personal learning and consultations with healthcare providers.

Awareness of potential interactions between herbal remedies and conventional medications is a critical safety consideration. Some herbs can potentiate or inhibit the effects of pharmaceuticals, leading to undesired outcomes. Before integrating herbal remedies into one's health regimen, discussing these plans with a healthcare professional, preferably one knowledgeable about both conventional and herbal medicine, is essential. This dialogue ensures that the use of herbs complements existing treatments and does not inadvertently compromise their efficacy or safety.

Recognizing that individual responses to herbal remedies can vary significantly is also key. Factors such as age, health status, and specific health conditions can influence how one's body reacts to a herb. What works harmoniously for one person may not be suitable for another, underscoring the importance of personalization in herbal medicine. Listening to one's body and observing any changes, whether beneficial or adverse, is fundamental to navigating the use of herbal remedies safely.

Finally, sourcing high-quality herbs is a practice that cannot be overstated. The purity, potency, and safety of herbal products can vary widely depending on the source. Opting for herbs and herbal products from reputable suppliers, ideally those who provide detailed information about the origin, cultivation practices, and processing of their products, helps ensure that the remedies are free from contaminants and adulterants that could compromise their safety and effectiveness.

In conclusion, embracing herbal remedies as a path to health and well-being is a journey that requires a commitment to safety, education, and mindful practice. By prioritizing accurate identification, understanding dosages, being aware of interactions, respecting individual responses, and sourcing quality herbs, beginners can confidently explore the world of herbal medicine. This approach not only maximizes the therapeutic potential of herbal remedies but also safeguards against the risks, making the journey towards natural healing both effective and enriching.

Part II: Herbal Materia Medica

Delving into the Herbal Materia Medica, we embark on a fascinating exploration of the medicinal plants that have been the cornerstone of natural healing practices for centuries. This compendium serves as a guide to the profound healing powers of herbs, offering insights into their properties, benefits, and uses. Each plant profiled here is a testament to nature's ability to foster health and wellness, providing a foundation for those seeking to integrate herbal remedies into their lives.

Aloe Vera, known for its soothing and healing properties, is a staple in natural skincare. Its gel, extracted from the leaves, offers relief for burns, wounds, and skin irritations, promoting healing and hydration. To harness Aloe Vera's benefits, simply apply the fresh gel directly to the affected area or look for products containing pure Aloe Vera.

Echinacea, a powerful immune booster, is revered for its ability to enhance the body's resistance to infections. Consuming Echinacea tea or tincture at the onset of cold or flu symptoms can support the immune system in fighting off these ailments. Start with a modest dose and consult a healthcare provider to ensure it complements your health regimen.

Lavender, celebrated for its calming and relaxing effects, is a balm for the nervous system. A few drops of Lavender essential oil in a diffuser can alleviate stress, promote relaxation, and improve sleep quality. Its versatility also extends to topical applications, where it can soothe minor burns and insect bites.

Peppermint, with its invigorating scent and properties, aids digestion and relieves headaches. A cup of Peppermint tea can ease digestive discomfort, while a diluted Peppermint oil applied to the temples may reduce headache severity. Always dilute essential oils with a carrier oil to avoid skin irritation.

Ginger, a potent anti-inflammatory and digestive aid, offers relief from nausea, indigestion, and inflammation. Incorporating fresh Ginger into meals or sipping on Ginger tea can harness its therapeutic benefits. For those new to Ginger, start with small amounts to gauge tolerance.

Turmeric, known for its anti-inflammatory and antioxidant properties, supports joint health and cardiovascular function. Adding Turmeric to your diet, whether as a spice in cooking or as a supplement, can provide health benefits. Combining Turmeric with black pepper enhances its absorption and effectiveness.

Milk Thistle, a liver tonic, supports detoxification and liver health. Its active compound, silymarin, has antioxidant properties that protect liver cells. Milk Thistle supplements can be a valuable addition to a detox regimen, but it's important to consult a healthcare provider before starting.

Chamomile, a gentle herb, promotes relaxation and sleep while soothing digestive issues. A cup of Chamomile tea before bed can improve sleep quality and ease gastrointestinal discomfort. Chamomile is generally safe, but those with allergies to plants in the daisy family should proceed with caution.

St. John's Wort, noted for its antidepressant effects, can support mood stabilization. However, it interacts with a wide range of medications, making it essential to consult with a healthcare professional before use. St. John's Wort can be taken as a tea, tincture, or supplement.

Dandelion, often considered a weed, is a nutritional powerhouse with detoxifying properties. Its leaves add a bitter yet beneficial element to salads, while the root can be brewed into a detoxifying tea. Dandelion supports liver function and digestion, showcasing the multifaceted nature of herbs.

Incorporating these herbs into your daily routine can open the door to enhanced health and well-being. However, it's crucial to approach herbal remedies with respect for their potency and potential interactions. Start with small doses, pay attention to your body's responses, and seek guidance from healthcare professionals, especially when combining herbs with conventional medications. By doing so, you can safely explore the rich world of herbal medicine, making informed choices that support your health journey.

Medicinal Plant Profiles

Aloe Vera emerges as a quintessential plant in the realm of natural healing with its profound soothing and hydrating abilities, particularly lauded for its efficacy in treating burns, cuts, and skin irritations. To leverage Aloe Vera's benefits, one can apply the gel directly from the leaf onto the affected area, ensuring immediate relief and acceleration in the healing process. This plant is not only a staple in topical treatments but also finds its place in enhancing digestive health when ingested in juice form, thanks to its internal soothing properties.

Echinacea stands out for its remarkable immune-boosting capabilities, making it a go-to herb during the cold and flu season. Its ability to enhance the body's immune response is harnessed through teas, tinctures, and supplements. Beginning with modest doses at the first sign of illness and consulting a healthcare provider for personalized advice ensures its optimal use.

Lavender, with its enchanting aroma, offers more than just a pleasant scent; it's a potent herb for alleviating stress, anxiety, and promoting restful sleep. Its essential oil, when used in a diffuser, can transform an environment, fostering relaxation and tranquility. Lavender's versatility extends to topical applications, providing relief from minor burns and insect bites, showcasing its anti-inflammatory and calming properties.

Peppermint, celebrated for its invigorating scent and digestive aid properties, is particularly effective in relieving gastrointestinal discomfort and headaches. A cup of peppermint tea can soothe an upset stomach, while a few drops of peppermint oil, diluted in a carrier oil and applied to the temples, can alleviate headache pain, demonstrating the herb's multifaceted uses.

Ginger, recognized for its potent anti-inflammatory and antioxidant properties, is a cornerstone in treating nausea, indigestion, and inflammatory conditions. Incorporating fresh ginger into one's diet or consuming ginger tea can unlock its therapeutic benefits, offering a natural remedy for a range of digestive issues.

Turmeric, with its vibrant color and health-promoting properties, is renowned for its anti-inflammatory and antioxidant effects, making it beneficial for joint health and overall wellness. Integrating turmeric into meals or taking it as a supplement, especially when combined with black pepper to enhance absorption, can yield significant health benefits.

Milk Thistle is lauded for its liver-protective qualities, with silymarin as its primary active compound, offering antioxidant and anti-inflammatory benefits that support liver detoxification processes. Supplements containing milk thistle can be a valuable addition to one's health regimen, particularly for those looking to support liver function.

Chamomile, with its gentle, soothing properties, is a treasure in promoting relaxation and sleep, alongside its benefits in digestive health. A cup of chamomile tea serves as a perfect nightcap, encouraging a restful night's sleep while easing digestive discomfort, making it a safe and effective herb for daily use.

St. John's Wort, known for its mood-stabilizing effects, is particularly beneficial for those dealing with mild to moderate depression. However, due to its interactions with various medications, consultation with a healthcare professional is paramount before incorporating it into one's health routine.

Dandelion, often overlooked as a common weed, is a powerhouse of nutrition and detoxification support. Its leaves can be used in salads for a nutritious boost, while the root makes a detoxifying tea, supporting liver function and aiding digestion, illustrating the diverse benefits of this ubiquitous plant.

By integrating these medicinal plants into daily life, individuals can harness the power of nature to enhance their health and well-being. Starting with small doses, observing the body's responses, and seeking professional guidance when combining herbs with conventional treatments ensures a safe and effective journey into the world of herbal medicine.

Comprehensive Guide to Medicinal Plants

Aloe Vera, a succulent plant, is renowned for its external healing properties, particularly for skin conditions like burns and cuts. Its gel, extracted from the leaves, can be applied topically to soothe and heal skin irritations, demonstrating its versatility as both a skincare remedy and a digestive aid when consumed in juice form.

Echinacea, distinguished by its coneflower appearance, plays a pivotal role in boosting the immune system. Its extracts are commonly used to prevent and treat the common cold, illustrating its effectiveness in enhancing the body's immune response. Incorporating Echinacea into your regimen at the onset of cold symptoms or as a preventive measure during flu season can bolster your immune defenses.

Lavender, with its fragrant purple flowers, is widely appreciated for its calming and relaxing effects. Utilizing Lavender essential oil in aromatherapy can alleviate stress, promote relaxation, and improve sleep quality. Additionally, Lavender oil can be applied to the skin to soothe minor burns, cuts, and insect bites, showcasing its anti-inflammatory properties.

Peppermint is celebrated for its digestive benefits, particularly in relieving symptoms of irritable bowel syndrome (IBS) and nausea. A cup of Peppermint tea can provide immediate relief for digestive discomfort, while Peppermint oil, when diluted and applied topically, can ease headache pain. This herb exemplifies the digestive and analgesic properties inherent in many medicinal plants.

Ginger, recognized for its potent anti-inflammatory and antioxidant effects, is a cornerstone in treating nausea and aiding digestion. Incorporating fresh Ginger or Ginger tea into your diet can leverage these therapeutic benefits, offering a natural remedy for a range of digestive issues and inflammation-related conditions.

Turmeric, known for its vibrant yellow color and health-promoting properties, is revered for its anti-inflammatory and antioxidant effects. Adding Turmeric to your diet, especially when combined with black pepper to enhance absorption, can provide significant health benefits, including joint health support and overall wellness enhancement.

Milk Thistle, with silymarin as its primary active compound, offers liver-protective qualities, supporting detoxification and liver health. Supplements containing Milk Thistle can be a valuable addition to a detox regimen, highlighting the importance of liver health in overall well-being.

Chamomile, a gentle herb, promotes relaxation and sleep while soothing digestive issues. Drinking Chamomile tea can improve sleep quality and ease gastrointestinal discomfort, making it a safe and effective herb for daily use, particularly for those seeking natural solutions for stress and digestive health.

St. John's Wort, recognized for its mood-stabilizing effects, is beneficial for those dealing with depression. However, due to its interactions with various medications, it's crucial to consult with a healthcare professional before use, emphasizing the importance of professional guidance in herbal supplementation.

Dandelion, often overlooked as a common weed, is a nutritional powerhouse with detoxifying properties. Incorporating Dandelion leaves into salads or brewing the root into tea can support liver function and aid digestion, showcasing the multifaceted nature of herbs in promoting health and wellness.

By understanding the properties, benefits, and uses of these medicinal plants, individuals can make informed decisions about incorporating herbal remedies into their health regimen. Starting with small doses, observing the body's responses, and seeking professional guidance when necessary, allows for a safe and effective exploration of herbal medicine. This guide serves as a foundational resource for those beginning their journey into the world of medicinal plants, offering a pathway to enhanced health and well-being through the power of nature.

Identification and Properties

Identifying and understanding the properties of medicinal plants is a foundational skill for anyone interested in herbal remedies. Each plant possesses a unique set of characteristics that determine its therapeutic value and how it should be used. This knowledge not only ensures the safety and efficacy of herbal remedies but also deepens one's connection to the natural world.

When identifying medicinal plants, the first step is to observe the physical attributes of the plant, including its leaves, flowers, stems, and roots. These features are crucial for distinguishing one plant from another and avoiding potentially harmful misidentifications. For example, the lance-shaped leaves and purple flowers of Echinacea purpurea distinguish it from other species, guiding its use for immune support.

Beyond physical identification, understanding a plant's properties involves learning about its active compounds and how they interact with the body. These properties can range from anti-inflammatory and antibacterial to sedative and diuretic. For instance, the presence of salicin in white willow bark contributes to its pain-relieving effects, similar to aspirin.

The habitat of a plant also plays a significant role in its identification and properties. Plants grown in their native environment tend to have stronger therapeutic qualities due to the optimal growing conditions. For example, the potency of ginseng, known for its adaptogenic properties, is influenced by the soil and climate conditions of its natural habitat.

Harvesting time is another critical factor that affects a plant's medicinal properties. Many plants have specific harvesting windows when their active compounds are at peak levels. For instance, harvesting calendula flowers in the morning after the dew has evaporated ensures the highest concentration of its soothing, anti-inflammatory compounds.

Safety is paramount when working with medicinal plants. While many herbs offer significant health benefits, they can also pose risks if not used correctly. Understanding the proper dosages, potential side effects, and contraindications of each plant is essential. For example, while St. John's Wort is beneficial for mild to moderate depression, it can interact with a wide range of medications and is not suitable for everyone.

In conclusion, the identification and understanding of medicinal plants' properties are crucial for anyone looking to incorporate herbal remedies into their health regimen. This knowledge ensures the safe and effective use of herbs, allowing individuals to harness the healing power of nature responsibly. Through careful study and observation, one can learn to recognize and utilize the unique gifts that each plant has to offer, contributing to a holistic approach to health and well-being.

Growing and Harvesting Herbs

Growing and harvesting your own herbs is an empowering step towards embracing a more holistic and natural lifestyle. It connects you with the cycle of nature and provides fresh, potent ingredients for your herbal remedies. To start, select a sunny spot in your garden or on a windowsill, as most herbs thrive in bright light. Begin with easy-to-grow herbs like basil, mint, and parsley, which don't require much space and can even flourish in pots, making them perfect for urban dwellers.

Preparation: involves choosing quality seeds or starter plants from reputable suppliers. Ensure your soil is well-draining and rich in organic matter. If using pots, select ones with adequate drainage holes and use a high-quality potting mix specifically designed for herbs.

Materials:

- Herb seeds or starter plants
- Compost or organic potting mix
- Mulch (optional, for outdoor gardens)

Tools:

- Trowel
- Watering can or hose with a gentle spray nozzle
- Pruners or scissors for harvesting

Safety measures: include wearing gloves to protect your hands while working with soil and sharp tools. Ensure proper labeling of your herbs to avoid confusion, especially when growing multiple varieties.

Step-by-step instructions:

1. Prepare your soil by loosening it and mixing in compost to improve fertility. If using pots, fill them with potting mix, leaving some space at the top.

2. Plant seeds or starter plants according to the instructions on the packet or tag. Generally, seeds should be planted at a depth twice their size.

3. Water gently but thoroughly after planting. Keep the soil consistently moist but not waterlogged.

4. As your herbs grow, thin seedlings if necessary to prevent overcrowding. This ensures adequate air circulation and reduces the risk of disease.

5. Apply mulch around outdoor plants to retain moisture, regulate soil temperature, and suppress weeds.

6. Begin harvesting when the plants are robust enough to recover from losing some leaves. Always harvest in the morning after the dew has evaporated for the best flavor.

7. To harvest, snip off leaves or stems with pruners or scissors, taking care not to remove more than one-third of the plant at a time to encourage further growth.

Cost estimate: Starting a small herb garden can cost as little as $20-$50, depending on whether you start from seeds or buy starter plants, and if you need to purchase pots and soil.

Time estimate: Initial setup of your herb garden can take a few hours. After that, expect to spend a few minutes daily on watering and regular maintenance such as weeding and checking for pests.

Safety tips:

- Label all herbs clearly, especially if you are growing varieties that look similar.

- Wash hands after handling soil or plants to prevent the spread of bacteria.

Troubleshooting:

- If your plants are not thriving, check to ensure they are getting enough light. Most herbs need at least 6 hours of direct sunlight daily.

- Yellowing leaves can indicate overwatering. Let the soil dry out slightly between waterings.

Maintenance: Regularly check your plants for pests and diseases. Pinch off any flowering buds to encourage leafier growth, as flowering can reduce the potency of the herbs.

Difficulty rating: ★☆☆☆☆ - Growing herbs is relatively easy, making it an excellent project for beginners.

Variations: Experiment with different herbs each season to discover what grows best in your climate and what flavors you enjoy most. Consider companion planting to naturally repel pests and enhance growth.

By growing your own herbs, you not only ensure a supply of fresh, organic ingredients for your remedies but also deepen your connection to the healing power of nature. Whether you're crafting a soothing tea or a healing salve, the herbs you've nurtured with your own hands carry a special potency and energy that can enhance their therapeutic benefits.

Part III: Herbal Preparation Techniques

Harvesting and preserving herbs are essential skills for anyone looking to utilize the natural healing properties of plants. The potency of herbal remedies is greatly influenced by how herbs are collected and stored, making it crucial to follow best practices to ensure the highest quality.

Objective: To effectively harvest and preserve herbs to maintain their medicinal properties for use in creating potent, healing remedies.

Preparation:

1. Identify the best time for harvesting each herb, as this varies significantly depending on the plant.

2. Gather all necessary materials and tools before beginning the harvesting process.

Materials:

- Gardening gloves

- Pruning shears or scissors

- Baskets or containers for collecting herbs

- Labels and markers

Tools:

- Dehydrator (optional)

- Oven (for low-temperature drying)

- Air-tight containers for storage

Safety measures: Wear gloves to protect your hands from cuts and potential skin irritants found on some plants. Ensure all tools are clean to prevent the introduction of pathogens to the herbs.

Step-by-step instructions:

1. **Harvesting**:

- Collect herbs early in the morning after the dew has evaporated but before the sun is too high. This is when their essential oils are most concentrated.

- Use pruning shears or scissors to cut herbs, taking care not to damage the plant or remove more than one-third of its growth.

- Select only the healthiest parts of the plant, avoiding any diseased or damaged leaves or stems.

2. **Drying**:

- Rinse herbs lightly to remove any dirt or insects, and pat dry with a towel.

- For air drying, tie herbs in small bundles and hang them upside down in a warm, dry, and well-ventilated area away from direct sunlight.

- To oven dry, place herbs on a baking sheet in a single layer and set the oven to the lowest possible temperature. Keep the oven door slightly open to allow moisture to escape. Check frequently to prevent burning.
- A dehydrator can also be used following the manufacturer's instructions for drying herbs.

3. **Storing**:
- Once completely dry, remove the leaves from the stems and store the herbs in air-tight containers. Glass jars with tight-fitting lids work well.
- Label each container with the herb's name and the date of storage.
- Store in a cool, dark place to preserve their potency.

Cost estimate: Minimal, primarily for storage containers if not already available. Costs can vary if a dehydrator is purchased, ranging from $30 to $300.

Time estimate: Harvesting can take a few hours depending on the quantity. Drying times vary: air drying may take 1-2 weeks, oven drying several hours, and dehydrator drying 1-24 hours based on the herb and method.

Safety tips:
- Always label herbs clearly during the drying and storage process to avoid confusion.
- Check stored herbs regularly for signs of mold or spoilage and discard any that are compromised.

Troubleshooting:
- If herbs mold while drying, it indicates too much moisture. Ensure better air circulation and lower humidity for the next batch.
- If herbs lose their color or scent quickly, they may have been over-dried or stored improperly. Adjust drying times and storage conditions accordingly.

Maintenance: Periodically check stored herbs for quality. Most dried herbs maintain potency for up to a year if stored correctly.

Difficulty rating: ★★☆☆☆ - Easy to moderate, depending on the chosen drying method and the scale of harvesting.

Variations: Experiment with different drying methods to find what works best for each herb type. Some herbs, like basil, may retain more flavor when frozen, offering an alternative preservation method.

By mastering these techniques, you can ensure that the herbs you use in remedies are as potent and effective as possible, bringing the full power of herbal healing into your home.

Harvesting and Preserving Herbs

Harvesting herbs at the right time ensures they are packed with the highest concentration of essential oils and active compounds, vital for their healing properties. The best time for harvesting most herbs is just before they flower, as this is when their energy is concentrated in the leaves, making them most potent. For annual herbs, this might mean harvesting in late spring or early summer, while perennials may be best harvested in the second year of growth, and always in the morning after the dew has evaporated but before the sun is too high. This timing helps preserve the natural oils and flavors that can be diminished by the sun's heat.

Materials:

- Clean, sharp scissors or pruning shears
- Baskets or containers for collecting herbs
- Labels and a permanent marker

Tools:

- Dehydrator or an oven
- Air-tight storage containers, preferably glass

Safety measures: Ensure all tools are clean and dry to prevent the introduction of mold or bacteria to the herbs. Wear gloves if you have sensitive skin or if handling herbs that could cause irritation.

Step-by-step instructions:

1. **Identify and Prepare**: Choose healthy, vibrant plants free from disease or damage. Early in the morning, gather your tools and prepare your collection baskets.

2. **Harvesting**: Using sharp scissors or pruning shears, cut the herbs, taking care not to damage the plant. Collect only the best specimens, avoiding any discolored or damaged parts.

3. **Rinsing (optional)**: Gently rinse the herbs if they are dusty or have soil on them. Pat them dry gently with a clean towel or let them air dry on paper towels.

4. **Drying**:

- **Air Drying**: Tie the herbs in small bundles and hang them upside down in a warm, dry place with good air circulation. Avoid direct sunlight as it can fade the colors and diminish the essential oils.

- **Oven Drying**: Preheat your oven to the lowest setting, spread the herbs on a baking sheet, and place them in the oven with the door slightly open to allow moisture to escape. Check frequently to ensure they do not burn.

- **Dehydrator**: Follow the manufacturer's instructions for drying herbs. This method is more controlled and can yield consistent results.

5. **Storing**: Once the herbs are completely dry, crumble the leaves and discard any stems. Store the dried herbs in air-tight containers, label them with the name and date, and keep them in a cool, dark place.

Cost estimate: Minimal, primarily for storage containers if not already on hand. Using existing kitchen appliances for drying eliminates the need for additional purchases.

Time estimate: Harvesting can take anywhere from a few minutes to an hour, depending on the size of your garden. Drying times vary from a few hours in a dehydrator or oven to several days or weeks for air drying.

Safety tips:
- Label all herbs during the drying and storage process to prevent any mix-ups.
- Check the dried herbs for any signs of mold or spoilage before storing.

Troubleshooting:
- If herbs mold during drying, it's likely due to insufficient air circulation or high humidity. Ensure a drier environment or try using a dehydrator.
- If herbs lose potency quickly, they may have been over-dried or exposed to too much light or heat during storage. Keep them in a cooler, darker place.

Maintenance: Check your stored herbs every few months for quality. Most will retain their potency for about a year if stored properly.

Difficulty rating: ★★☆☆☆ - Relatively easy with attention to detail required for best results.

Variations: Experiment with different drying and storage methods to find what best preserves the flavors and medicinal qualities of each herb. Some herbs may also be preserved by freezing or in oil, offering alternative methods for maintaining their potency.

Best Practices for Harvesting

Harvesting herbs at the right time and in the correct manner is crucial for maximizing their medicinal properties and ensuring the longevity of your plants. To begin, always harvest herbs in the morning after the dew has evaporated but before the sun is high. This is when the plants' essential oils are at their peak, offering the most potent medicinal qualities. Use sharp, clean scissors or pruning shears to make clean cuts, which help prevent damage to the plant and reduce the risk of disease.

For leaves, the best time to harvest is before the plant flowers, as this is when the leaves contain the highest concentration of active compounds. However, if you are harvesting flowers, wait until they are fully open but not wilted. Roots should be harvested in the fall when the plant's energy is concentrated below ground. Annuals can be pulled up by the root, while perennials should be carefully dug up to preserve the plant.

Drying is the most common method for preserving herbs, and it's important to do this correctly to maintain their medicinal properties. Tie harvested herbs in small bundles and hang them upside down in a warm, dry, and well-ventilated area out of direct sunlight. Alternatively, herbs can be laid out on a screen or rack. Check on them regularly, and once they are completely dry, usually within a week or two, remove the leaves from the stems and store them in airtight containers labeled with the date of harvest.

When harvesting, only take about one-third of the plant material at a time to ensure the plant remains healthy and can continue to grow. It's also important to be mindful of the plant's growth cycle and only harvest when there is enough plant material to sustain growth. Overharvesting can weaken or even kill the plant, so always harvest responsibly.

Remember to leave some flowers on the plant if you are harvesting before the plant has gone to seed, as this allows the plant to complete its life cycle and reseed for the next year. Additionally, consider the environmental impact of your harvesting practices. Harvesting wild plants should be done with care to avoid depleting natural populations. Always ensure that you have correctly identified the plant and that it is not endangered or protected.

By following these best practices for harvesting, you can ensure that you are collecting the highest quality material for your herbal remedies while also respecting and preserving the plants and their natural habitat. This mindful approach to harvesting not only benefits your health and well-being but also supports the sustainability and resilience of the plant communities you rely on.

Drying and Storing Herbs

After harvesting your herbs, the next crucial steps are drying and storing them to preserve their medicinal properties and flavors. Drying herbs effectively removes moisture, inhibiting the growth of bacteria and mold, ensuring that your herbs retain their potency for use in remedies and teas.

Objective: To dry and store herbs maintaining their quality and potency.

Preparation:

1. Gather harvested herbs, ensuring they are clean and free from pests.

2. Select a dry, warm, and well-ventilated area out of direct sunlight for drying.

Materials:

- Freshly harvested herbs

- String or rubber bands (for bundling)

- Paper bags (optional)

- Airtight containers

Tools:

- Scissors or garden shears

- Labels and marker

Safety measures: Ensure the area is free from dust and pets to maintain cleanliness.

Step-by-step instructions:

1. **Bundle and Hang:** Tie small bundles of herbs with string or rubber bands. Hang them upside down in your chosen area. For herbs with smaller leaves, you can cover them with paper bags to protect from dust, poking holes in the bag for ventilation.

2. **Screen Drying:** Alternatively, lay herbs out on a screen or rack in a single layer for more airflow. This method is ideal for herbs that might lose their leaves when hung.

3. **Check Regularly:** Depending on the humidity and temperature, herbs can take 1-2 weeks to dry completely. Check them every few days to ensure they are drying evenly and to prevent mold.

4. **Storage:** Once herbs are fully dried, gently remove the leaves from the stems and transfer them to airtight containers. Glass jars or metal tins are ideal. Ensure containers are labeled with the herb name and date of storage.

5. **Location:** Store your containers in a cool, dark place to preserve the herbs' essential oils and medicinal properties.

Cost estimate: Minimal, primarily for containers if not already available.

Time estimate: 1-2 weeks for drying, depending on conditions.

Safety tips:

- Ensure herbs are completely dry before storage to prevent mold.

- Keep drying herbs away from kitchens or bathrooms to avoid moisture.

Troubleshooting:

- If herbs aren't drying evenly, rotate or rearrange them for better airflow.

- If mold appears, discard affected parts immediately to prevent it from spreading.

Maintenance: Periodically check stored herbs for quality. Properly dried and stored herbs can last up to a year.

Difficulty rating: ★☆☆☆☆

By following these steps, you'll ensure your herbs are preserved at their peak potency for your herbal remedies, teas, and culinary uses, empowering you to leverage the natural benefits of herbs year-round.

Creating Herbal Remedies

Creating herbal remedies at home is a rewarding way to take control of your health and well-being. This process allows you to harness the natural healing properties of plants in a form that suits your needs, whether it's for soothing a sore throat, calming an upset stomach, or easing stress. The key to successful herbal remedy creation is understanding the basic methods of preparation, which include making teas, tinctures, salves, and capsules. Each method extracts the medicinal properties of herbs in different ways, suitable for various uses and conditions.

Objective: To create effective, safe, and personalized herbal remedies at home.

Preparation:

1. Identify the health issue or condition you wish to address.

2. Select the appropriate herbs based on their medicinal properties.

3. Choose the most suitable form of remedy (tea, tincture, salve, or capsule).

Materials:

- Selected herbs

- Alcohol (for tinctures) or oil (for salves)

- Capsules (if making herbal capsules)

- Beeswax (if making salves)

- Glass jars or bottles

- Cheesecloth or fine mesh strainer

Tools:

- Teapot or saucepan

- Measuring cups and spoons

- Grinder (for herbs and making powders)

- Small funnel

- Double boiler (for salves)

Safety measures:

- Always source high-quality, organic herbs.

- Ensure all tools and containers are clean to prevent contamination.

- Label all remedies with ingredients and the date of creation.

Step-by-step instructions:

1. **Teas:** Place one tablespoon of dried herbs or two tablespoons of fresh herbs per cup of boiling water. Steep for 10-15 minutes, strain, and enjoy. Teas are best for immediate use.

2. **Tinctures:** Fill a glass jar ⅔ with dried herbs, then cover completely with alcohol. Seal the jar and store in a cool, dark place for 4-6 weeks, shaking daily. Strain the liquid through cheesecloth into a clean bottle. Tinctures are concentrated and long-lasting.

3. **Salves:** Gently heat one cup of oil infused with your chosen herbs in a double boiler, then stir in ¼ cup of beeswax until melted. Pour into small containers and let cool. Salves are excellent for topical application.

4. **Capsules:** Grind dried herbs into a fine powder. Using a small funnel, fill empty capsules with the powder. Capsules are convenient for precise dosages and portability.

Cost estimate: Varies depending on the herbs and materials used but generally low to moderate.

Time estimate: Preparation time varies by remedy type, ranging from 15 minutes for teas to 6 weeks for tinctures.

Safety tips:

- Test a small amount of any new remedy to check for adverse reactions.

- Consult with a healthcare provider before using herbal remedies, especially if pregnant, nursing, or taking medication.

Troubleshooting:

- If a tincture is too strong, dilute it with water.

- If a salve is too hard, remelt and add more oil; if too soft, add more beeswax.

Maintenance: Store remedies in a cool, dark place. Most will last for up to a year if properly stored.

Difficulty rating: ★☆☆☆☆ to ★★☆☆☆, depending on the remedy type.

Variations: Experiment with combining herbs to address multiple symptoms or to create a more pleasant flavor.

By following these steps, even beginners can create their own herbal remedies tailored to their health needs and preferences. This hands-on approach not only empowers you to take an active role in your health care but also deepens your connection to the natural world. Whether you're soothing a cough with a homemade syrup or easing a headache with a lavender tincture, the art of making herbal remedies is a valuable skill for anyone looking to enhance their well-being naturally.

Making Tinctures and Extracts

Making tinctures and extracts is a fundamental skill for anyone interested in harnessing the potent healing properties of herbs. These concentrated forms of herbal medicine offer a convenient and effective way to preserve and utilize the active compounds found in plants. This guide will walk you through the simple steps to create your own tinctures and extracts at home, ensuring you have access to natural remedies year-round.

Objective: To prepare homemade tinctures and extracts that capture the essence and therapeutic benefits of herbs.

Preparation:

- Decide on the herb or combination of herbs you wish to use based on the health benefits you're seeking.

- Research and source high-quality, organic herbs to ensure the purity and potency of your tincture or extract.

Materials:

- Dried or fresh herbs

- High-proof alcohol (for tinctures) or vinegar/glycerin (for non-alcoholic extracts)

- Glass jar with a tight-fitting lid

- Dark glass bottles for storage

- Label and marker

Tools:

- Measuring cups and spoons

- Fine mesh strainer or cheesecloth

- Funnel

- Grinder (optional, for breaking down dried herbs)

Safety measures:

- Ensure your workspace is clean to avoid contamination.

- Label your tinctures clearly, including the date and ingredients.

Step-by-step instructions:

1. **Prepare Your Herbs:** If using dried herbs, grind them coarsely to increase the surface area for extraction. For fresh herbs, chop them finely.

2. **Fill Your Jar:** Place your herbs in the glass jar, filling it halfway for dried herbs or three-quarters for fresh herbs.

3. **Add Your Solvent:** Pour the alcohol or alternative solvent over the herbs, completely covering them by at least two inches. If using fresh herbs, ensure the solvent accounts for the water content of the herbs by filling the jar to nearly full.

4. **Seal and Store:** Tighten the lid on your jar and shake it gently to mix the herbs and solvent. Label your jar with the date and ingredients. Store the jar in a cool, dark place.

5. **Wait:** Let the mixture sit for 4-6 weeks, shaking it daily to help the extraction process.

6. **Strain:** After the waiting period, strain the liquid through a fine mesh strainer or cheesecloth into a clean bowl. Compress the herbs to squeeze out as much liquid as possible.

7. **Bottle:** Using a funnel, transfer the strained liquid into dark glass bottles. Label each bottle with the herb, date, and type of solvent used.

8. **Store:** Keep your tinctures and extracts in a cool, dark place. Alcohol-based tinctures can last for several years, while vinegar or glycerin-based extracts should be used within a year.

Cost estimate: Low to moderate, depending on the cost of herbs and alcohol or alternative solvents.

Time estimate: 4-6 weeks for maceration, plus preparation and bottling time.

Safety tips:

- Always use food-grade alcohol or solvents.

- Be mindful of any allergies or sensitivities to the herbs you're using.

Troubleshooting:

- If mold develops, this indicates contamination. Discard the tincture and start over with sterilized equipment.

- If the tincture is too weak, allow it to macerate for a longer period, or consider adding more herbs at the start of the process.

Maintenance: Check the bottles periodically for any signs of spoilage or degradation. Ensure the lids are tightly sealed to prevent evaporation.

Difficulty rating: ★☆☆☆☆

Variations: Experiment with different herbs and combinations to tailor the health benefits to your needs. Non-alcoholic extracts can be made using glycerin or vinegar, offering alternatives for those avoiding alcohol.

By mastering the art of making tinctures and extracts, you empower yourself to create personalized, natural remedies that support your health and well-being. This process not only connects you with the age-old tradition of herbal medicine but also provides you with tools to care for yourself and your family in a more holistic and informed way.

Crafting Salves and Ointments

Crafting salves and ointments is an essential skill for anyone looking to harness the healing power of herbs in a form that's convenient and versatile for topical application. These preparations are ideal for addressing a wide range of skin issues, from dryness and irritation to cuts and bruises, providing a protective barrier that aids in the skin's natural healing process. The process of making your own salves and ointments allows for customization of ingredients to target specific concerns, ensuring you have a remedy on hand that is tailored to your needs or those of your family.

Objective: To create herbal salves and ointments that soothe, heal, and protect the skin using natural ingredients.

Preparation:

1. Choose herbs based on their healing properties. For example, calendula for healing wounds, lavender for soothing skin, or arnica for reducing inflammation.

2. Decide on a base for your salve or ointment. Options include oils like olive, coconut, or almond oil, and beeswax or shea butter as a thickening agent.

Materials:

- Dried or fresh herbs
- Carrier oil (olive, coconut, almond)
- Beeswax or shea butter
- Essential oils (optional, for added therapeutic benefits or fragrance)
- Glass jars or metal tins for storage

Tools:

- Double boiler or a small pot and heat-safe bowl
- Fine mesh strainer or cheesecloth
- Measuring cups and spoons
- Stirring utensil

- Funnel (optional, for transferring liquid)

Safety measures:

- Ensure all tools and containers are thoroughly cleaned to prevent contamination.

- Be cautious when handling hot oils and beeswax to avoid burns.

Step-by-step instructions:

1. **Infuse the Oil:** Place your chosen herbs in a double boiler and cover with your carrier oil. Gently heat the herbs and oil over low heat for 2-3 hours to allow the medicinal properties of the herbs to infuse into the oil. Avoid overheating to preserve the beneficial qualities of the oil.

2. **Strain the Oil:** After infusion, remove from heat and let cool slightly. Strain the oil through a fine mesh strainer or cheesecloth into a clean bowl, pressing the herbs to extract as much oil as possible.

3. **Add Beeswax or Shea Butter:** Return the strained oil to the double boiler and add beeswax or shea butter. Use about 1 ounce of beeswax per cup of infused oil for a standard salve consistency. Adjust the amount for a softer or firmer salve as desired.

4. **Melt and Mix:** Heat gently, stirring until the beeswax or shea butter is completely melted and the mixture is well combined.

5. **Add Essential Oils:** Once melted, remove from heat and stir in any essential oils if using, usually a few drops per ounce of salve mixture.

6. **Pour into Containers:** Quickly pour the mixture into your prepared jars or tins before it begins to set. Use a funnel if necessary to avoid spills.

7. **Cool and Set:** Allow the salves to cool and solidify at room temperature. This may take several hours. Avoid moving the containers until the salves are fully set.

8. **Label:** Label your containers with the ingredients and date made for future reference.

Cost estimate: Low to moderate, depending on the cost of ingredients selected.

Time estimate: Approximately 3-4 hours, including infusion and cooling time.

Safety tips:

- Test a small amount of the finished salve on the skin to ensure there is no adverse reaction before widespread use.

- Keep salves in a cool, dark place to prolong shelf life.

Troubleshooting:

- If the salve is too soft, remelt and add more beeswax. If too hard, remelt and add more oil.

- If separation occurs, remelt the salve, ensuring thorough mixing before setting again.

Maintenance: Store salves in a cool, dark place. Most homemade salves can last for up to a year if stored properly.

Difficulty rating: ★★☆☆☆

Variations: Experiment with different herb and oil combinations to create salves for various purposes, such as a peppermint and eucalyptus salve for respiratory issues or a tea tree and neem oil salve for fungal infections.

By mastering the art of crafting salves and ointments, you gain the ability to create personalized, natural remedies that soothe, heal, and protect the skin. This skill not only empowers you to care for your family's skin health in a more holistic way but also connects you with the age-old practice of herbal medicine, utilizing the gifts of nature to support healing and well-being.

Herbal Teas and Infusions

Herbal teas and infusions are a cornerstone of natural healing, offering a gentle yet effective way to harness the therapeutic properties of herbs. These beverages not only provide hydration but also deliver the health benefits of various plants directly to your system. Whether you're seeking to calm a troubled stomach, ease stress, or boost your immune system, there's an herbal tea or infusion that can help.

Objective: To prepare and enjoy herbal teas and infusions that promote health and wellness.

Preparation:

1. Choose your herb or blend of herbs based on the desired health benefits.

2. Measure the appropriate amount of herb(s) needed for your tea or infusion.

Materials:

- Fresh or dried herbs

- Boiling water

- Tea infuser or teapot

- Measuring spoons

- Cups or mugs

Tools:

- Kettle or pot for boiling water

- Strainer (if not using an infuser or teapot with one built-in)

Safety measures:

- Ensure herbs are correctly identified and sourced from reputable suppliers to avoid contamination.

- Be aware of any personal allergies to specific herbs.

Step-by-step instructions:

1. **Boil Water:** Begin by boiling water in a kettle or pot. For most herbal teas, use one cup (8 ounces) of water per serving.

2. **Measure Herbs:** Use one teaspoon of dried herbs or two teaspoons of fresh herbs per cup of boiling water. Adjust according to taste and the herb's strength.

3. **Steep:** Place the herbs in the tea infuser or directly into the teapot. Pour boiling water over the herbs and cover to steep. For a stronger infusion, cover and steep for 10-15 minutes. For a milder tea, steep for 5-7 minutes.

4. **Strain:** If you've placed the herbs directly in the pot or cup, strain the tea into another cup to remove the herb particles. If using an infuser, simply remove it from the cup or pot.

5. **Enjoy:** Sip your herbal tea or infusion while it's warm. Sweeten with honey or lemon if desired.

Cost estimate: Minimal, especially if using herbs grown in your own garden.

Time estimate: 15-20 minutes from boiling water to enjoying your tea.

Safety tips:

- Always start with a small amount of any new herb to ensure you do not have an adverse reaction.

- Consult with a healthcare provider if you are pregnant, nursing, or on medication before adding new herbal teas to your regimen.

Troubleshooting:

- If the tea is too strong, dilute it with more boiling water.

- If the tea is too weak, add more herbs and steep for a longer time.

Maintenance: Store dried herbs in a cool, dark place in airtight containers to maintain their potency.

Difficulty rating: ★☆☆☆☆

Variations: Experiment with blending different herbs to create your own unique flavors and health benefits. Common blends include chamomile and lavender for relaxation, peppermint and ginger for digestion, or echinacea and elderberry for immune support.

By incorporating herbal teas and infusions into your daily routine, you can enjoy the myriad health benefits they offer. Whether used for specific health concerns or simply for relaxation and enjoyment, herbal teas are a simple, enjoyable way to support your overall well-being.

Herbal Capsules and Pills

Herbal capsules and pills provide a convenient and precise way to incorporate the benefits of herbs into your daily routine. This method of herbal remedy is especially appealing for those who are often on the go or may not enjoy the taste of herbal teas and tinctures. Capsules and pills offer the advantage of exact dosages and ease of transport, making it simpler to maintain consistency in your herbal wellness regimen.

Objective: To create your own herbal capsules and pills, allowing for personalized, convenient, and precise herbal supplementation.

Preparation:

1. Decide on the herbal blend or single herb you wish to encapsulate, considering your health goals.

2. Research the herbs to ensure they are safe for you to use and compatible with any medications or conditions you have.

Materials:

- Dried herbs, finely ground

- Empty capsules

- Capsule filling machine (optional but helpful for larger batches)

Tools:

- Grinder (coffee grinder works well for this purpose)

- Small bowl

- Spatula or small spoon

- Gloves (optional, for cleanliness)

Safety measures:

- Source high-quality, organic herbs to avoid contaminants.

- Ensure your workspace and tools are clean to prevent contamination.

- Wear gloves to keep the process sanitary, especially if preparing capsules for others.

Step-by-step instructions:

1. **Grind the Herbs:** Use a grinder to finely powder your chosen herbs. This increases the surface area, making it easier to fill capsules and ensuring better absorption in the body.

2. **Set Up the Capsule Machine:** If using a capsule filling machine, set it up according to the manufacturer's instructions. These machines typically come with a base for holding the bottom halves of the capsules, a top for the capsule caps, and a tamper for packing the herbs.

3. **Fill the Capsules:** Whether using a machine or not, the next step is to fill the empty capsules with your powdered herbs. If doing this by hand, open each capsule and use a small spoon or spatula

to pack the herb powder tightly into the bottom half of the capsule, then cap it with the top half. If using a machine, follow the instructions to fill multiple capsules at once.

4. **Seal the Capsules:** Some capsules snap together, while others might require a slight twist. Ensure each capsule is securely closed to prevent the powder from spilling out.

5. **Store the Capsules:** Transfer the filled capsules to a clean, dry container. Label the container with the herb name, date of creation, and dosage if known.

Cost estimate: Low to moderate, depending on the volume of herbs and whether you choose to invest in a capsule machine.

Time estimate: 1-2 hours, depending on the quantity of capsules being made and whether a filling machine is used.

Safety tips:

- Consult with a healthcare provider before beginning any new herbal regimen, especially if you have existing health conditions or are taking medications.

- Start with a small dosage to ensure you do not have an adverse reaction to the herb.

Troubleshooting:

- If the powder is not packing well into the capsules, ensure it is finely ground. A coarser grind can make the process more difficult.

- If capsules are not closing properly, check to ensure no powder is caught in the rim of the capsule.

Maintenance: Store your capsules in a cool, dark place to preserve their potency. Most herbal capsules will remain potent for up to a year if stored properly.

Difficulty rating: ★★☆☆☆

Variations: Experiment with creating blends of herbs to target specific health concerns. For example, a blend of ginger, turmeric, and black pepper can be made into capsules for natural inflammation support.

Creating your own herbal capsules and pills not only allows for a customized approach to herbal supplementation but also empowers you to take control of your health in a more hands-on way. With the right preparation and materials, you can easily incorporate the ancient wisdom of herbs into your modern lifestyle, ensuring that you're getting the precise, targeted support you need for your health and wellness goals.

Part IV: Remedies for Common Ailments

Addressing common ailments with herbal remedies provides a natural path to healing that aligns with the body's rhythms and the wisdom of nature. From digestive issues to respiratory health, the power of plants offers gentle yet effective solutions. This part delves into creating herbal remedies that target these widespread concerns, empowering you with the knowledge to craft your own natural medicines at home.

Digestive Health: A harmonious digestive system is crucial for overall well-being, yet many suffer from common complaints such as indigestion, bloating, and nausea. Herbal remedies can offer significant relief. For instance, peppermint tea is renowned for its ability to soothe an upset stomach and improve digestion. To prepare, steep one teaspoon of dried peppermint leaves in one cup of boiling water for ten minutes. Strain and enjoy up to three times a day. Similarly, ginger, with its potent anti-inflammatory properties, can be used to alleviate nausea. A simple ginger tea made by simmering slices of fresh ginger root in water for fifteen minutes can be sipped throughout the day to provide relief.

Respiratory Health: Herbs also play a pivotal role in supporting respiratory health, offering relief from colds, coughs, and asthma. A time-honored remedy for coughs is thyme tea, which possesses antibacterial and antiviral properties. Combine one teaspoon of dried thyme with a cup of boiling water, steep for ten minutes, then strain. Drinking this tea several times a day can help ease cough symptoms. Elderberry syrup is another powerful tool in the herbal arsenal against respiratory infections, known for its immune-boosting capabilities. Making your own elderberry syrup involves simmering elderberries with water and honey to create a thick, sweet concoction that can be taken daily during cold and flu season.

Skin and Hair Care: The skin, our largest organ, and our hair, often referred to as our crowning glory, can also benefit from herbal treatments. Calendula, with its soothing and healing properties, can be infused into a salve for treating dry skin, rashes, and minor cuts. To create a calendula salve, gently heat dried calendula petals in a carrier oil such as coconut or almond oil, strain, then mix with melted beeswax until the desired consistency is reached. For hair care, rosemary can stimulate growth and add shine. A simple rosemary hair rinse can be made by steeping rosemary leaves in boiling water, then cooling and straining the mixture before applying it to the hair after shampooing.

Pain and Inflammation: Chronic pain and inflammation can significantly impact quality of life, but herbs like turmeric and willow bark offer natural pain relief without the side effects associated with over-the-counter medications. Turmeric, known for its curcumin content, can be incorporated into daily meals or taken as a supplement. Willow bark, often referred to as "nature's aspirin," can be brewed into a tea by simmering the bark in water for 10-15 minutes. This tea can then be consumed in moderation to alleviate pain and reduce inflammation.

In creating these remedies, it's crucial to source high-quality, organic herbs and to be mindful of dosages and potential interactions with medications. Always start with small amounts to see how your body responds, and consult with a healthcare provider if you have any concerns or pre-existing conditions. By integrating these herbal solutions into your health care routine, you can harness the natural power of plants to address common ailments, enhancing your well-being and leading a more holistic lifestyle.

Urinary Tract Health: Herbal remedies can be a boon for those suffering from urinary tract infections (UTIs) and discomfort. Cranberry is widely recognized for its ability to prevent and aid in the treatment of UTIs due to its proanthocyanidins that prevent bacteria from adhering to the urinary tract walls. For a preventive measure, consuming unsweetened cranberry juice daily can be beneficial. Additionally, uva-ursi, also known as bearberry, has antiseptic properties and can be taken as a tea to help cleanse the urinary tract. To prepare, steep one teaspoon of dried uva-ursi leaves in one cup of boiling water for about 10 minutes, strain, and drink up to two times a day. Note, it's important to use uva-ursi with caution and not for prolonged periods as it can have side effects and is not recommended during pregnancy.

Sleep and Relaxation: A good night's sleep is foundational to health, yet many struggle with insomnia and restlessness. Herbs like valerian root and chamomile are well-known for their calming and sedative properties. Valerian root can be taken as a capsule or as a tea before bedtime to promote sleep. For chamomile tea, steep two to three teaspoons of dried chamomile flowers in one cup of boiling water for 10-15 minutes, then strain and drink before bedtime for a restful sleep. Adding lavender to a bath or as an essential oil diffused in the bedroom can also enhance relaxation and improve sleep quality.

Heart Health: Hawthorn berry has been traditionally used to support heart health, with research suggesting it can improve cardiovascular function. Hawthorn can be consumed as a tea, tincture, or capsule to help regulate blood pressure and support the heart. To make hawthorn tea, steep one teaspoon of dried hawthorn berries in one cup of boiling water for 15 minutes, strain, and enjoy. It's a gentle remedy, but as with any herb that affects heart health, it's wise to consult with a healthcare provider before starting.

Mental Clarity and Focus: In the modern world, maintaining mental clarity and focus can be challenging. Ginkgo biloba is renowned for its ability to improve cognitive function. It increases blood flow to the brain, which can help with memory and focus. Ginkgo leaves can be taken in capsule form or as a tea. For the tea, steep one teaspoon of dried ginkgo leaves in a cup of boiling water for about 10 minutes, strain, and drink. Since ginkgo can interact with certain medications, including blood thinners, it's important to consult with a healthcare professional before adding it to your regimen.

Joint Health: For those dealing with arthritis and joint pain, herbs like ginger and turmeric can offer natural relief due to their anti-inflammatory properties. Incorporating ginger and turmeric into your diet, either fresh, in capsules, or as a tea, can help reduce inflammation and pain. A simple tea can be made by simmering slices of fresh ginger and turmeric root in water for 15 minutes, straining, and drinking warm. Adding black pepper can enhance the absorption of turmeric's active compound, curcumin, increasing its effectiveness.

By incorporating these herbal remedies into your daily routine, you can naturally support your body's health across a variety of systems. Remember, while herbs offer incredible health benefits, they should be used responsibly and in conjunction with advice from healthcare professionals, especially if you have pre-existing conditions or are taking medications. Embracing the power of herbs can lead to a more balanced, healthful life, empowering you to take control of your well-being in harmony with nature's gifts.

Digestive Health

Peppermint, renowned for its soothing properties, offers a natural remedy for digestive discomforts such as indigestion and bloating. To harness these benefits, a simple peppermint tea can be prepared by steeping one teaspoon of dried peppermint leaves in one cup of boiling water for ten minutes. This tea can be consumed up to three times daily to aid digestion and relieve discomfort.

Ginger, another powerful herb, is celebrated for its anti-inflammatory properties and its ability to alleviate nausea. A ginger tea can be made by simmering slices of fresh ginger root in water for fifteen minutes. Drinking this tea throughout the day can provide relief from nausea and promote digestive health.

For those experiencing bloating and gas, fennel seeds offer relief due to their antispasmodic and gas-relieving properties. A fennel seed tea can be made by crushing one teaspoon of fennel seeds and steeping them in boiling water for ten minutes. Consuming this tea can help ease bloating and digestive spasms.

Chamomile tea, known for its calming effects, can also benefit the digestive system by soothing the gastrointestinal tract and reducing inflammation. Prepare chamomile tea by steeping two to three teaspoons of dried chamomile flowers in one cup of boiling water for 10-15 minutes, then strain and enjoy before bedtime or any time discomfort is experienced.

Dandelion root tea acts as a gentle liver tonic and digestive aid. Simmer one teaspoon of dried dandelion root in water for 15 minutes to make a tea that supports digestion and detoxification processes within the body.

To incorporate these herbal remedies into daily routines, consider the following steps:

1. Identify the specific digestive issue you are experiencing, such as indigestion, bloating, nausea, or general discomfort.

2. Select the appropriate herb based on its medicinal properties that address your specific digestive needs.

3. Prepare the herbal tea using the guidelines provided for each herb, ensuring to steep the herbs for the recommended amount of time to extract their beneficial properties.

4. Consume the herbal tea at the recommended frequency, paying attention to how your body responds to the remedy.

It's important to source high-quality, organic herbs to ensure the purity and potency of your digestive remedies. Additionally, always start with small amounts to monitor your body's response, and consult with a healthcare provider if you have any concerns or pre-existing conditions. By integrating these herbal solutions into your healthcare routine, you can support your digestive health naturally and effectively.

1. *Ginger Tea for Nausea*

Beneficial effects: Ginger tea is renowned for its ability to alleviate nausea, making it an excellent remedy for indigestion, morning sickness, and motion sickness. Its natural compounds, such as gingerol, have anti-inflammatory and antioxidant properties that can help soothe the stomach and improve digestive health.

Ingredients:

- 1 inch fresh ginger root, thinly sliced
- 2 cups water
- Honey to taste (optional)
- Lemon slice for garnish (optional)

Instructions:

1. Peel and thinly slice the fresh ginger root.
2. In a saucepan, bring 2 cups of water to a boil.
3. Add the sliced ginger to the boiling water.
4. Reduce the heat and simmer for 10-15 minutes, depending on how strong you prefer the tea.
5. Strain the tea into a mug, removing the ginger slices.
6. Add honey to taste, if desired.
7. Garnish with a slice of lemon for an extra boost of flavor and vitamin C.

Variations:

- For a cold remedy, add a pinch of ground cinnamon or turmeric to the tea while it simmers.
- If you prefer a caffeine kick, steep a bag of green tea with the ginger.
- For additional digestive benefits, include a few fennel seeds or a stick of cinnamon with the ginger.

Storage tips:

- Fresh ginger can be stored in the refrigerator for up to three weeks or in the freezer for up to six months for longer preservation.
- Prepared ginger tea can be stored in the refrigerator for up to two days. Reheat gently on the stove or enjoy cold.

Tips for allergens:

- Ginger tea is naturally free from common allergens such as gluten, dairy, and nuts, making it a safe choice for most people. However, always ensure that any added ingredients (such as honey or lemon) are also allergen-free for your needs.

Scientific references:

- "Ginger in gastrointestinal disorders: A systematic review of clinical trials," published in Food Science & Nutrition, highlights ginger's effectiveness in treating nausea and digestive issues.
- "Anti-Oxidative and Anti-Inflammatory Effects of Ginger in Health and Physical Activity: Review of Current Evidence," published in the International Journal of Preventive Medicine, supports ginger's health benefits, including its anti-nausea properties.

2. Peppermint Oil Capsules

Beneficial effects: Peppermint oil capsules are renowned for their ability to soothe digestive issues, including indigestion, bloating, and nausea. They work by relaxing the muscles of your stomach, reducing the pain associated with gas and spasms, and promoting overall digestive health. Additionally, peppermint oil has antimicrobial properties that can help in managing intestinal discomfort caused by bacteria.

Ingredients:

- 0.2 ml (about 4 drops) of food-grade peppermint oil

- Empty vegetarian or gelatin capsules (size 0 or 00)

Instructions:

1. Carefully open an empty capsule by gently pulling apart the two halves.

2. Using a dropper, add approximately 4 drops (0.2 ml) of food-grade peppermint oil into the larger half of the capsule.

3. Reconnect the two halves of the capsule to seal the peppermint oil inside.

4. Repeat the process for the desired number of capsules.

5. Store the prepared capsules in a cool, dry place away from direct sunlight.

Storage tips:

Keep the capsules in a small, airtight container to protect them from moisture and light. If stored properly, the capsules should remain potent and effective for up to a month.

Tips for allergens: For those with dietary restrictions or allergies, ensure that the empty capsules you use are compatible with your needs. Vegetarian capsules are a great alternative for individuals avoiding animal products.

Scientific references:

Studies have shown that peppermint oil is effective in relieving symptoms of irritable bowel syndrome (IBS), including indigestion, bloating, and gas. One such study published in the "Journal of Clinical Gastroenterology" found that patients who took peppermint oil capsules for four weeks reported significant improvements in IBS symptoms compared to those who took a placebo.

3. Fennel Seed Infusion

Beneficial effects: Fennel Seed Infusion is renowned for its ability to alleviate digestive discomforts such as indigestion, bloating, and nausea. The active compounds in fennel seeds, including anethole, fenchone, and estragole, have antispasmodic and anti-inflammatory properties that can relax the muscles in the gastrointestinal tract, facilitating smoother digestion and relieving gas and bloating.

Ingredients:

- 1 teaspoon of fennel seeds

- 1 cup of boiling water

Instructions:

1. Crush the fennel seeds lightly with a mortar and pestle to release their oils.

2. Place the crushed seeds in a teapot or a cup.

3. Pour one cup of boiling water over the fennel seeds.

4. Cover and steep for 10 to 15 minutes.

5. Strain the infusion into a cup.

6. Drink the warm fennel seed infusion slowly.

Variations:

- For a sweeter taste, add a teaspoon of honey or a slice of fresh ginger for added digestive benefits.

- Combine with peppermint leaves or chamomile flowers for a soothing blend that further enhances digestive relief.

Storage tips: Store unused fennel seeds in a cool, dark place in an airtight container to maintain their potency and freshness. The prepared fennel seed infusion should be consumed fresh, but can be refrigerated for up to 24 hours if necessary. Reheat gently without boiling to enjoy later.

Tips for allergens:

Individuals with allergies to celery or carrots, which are in the same family as fennel, should proceed with caution when trying fennel seed infusion for the first time. Always start with a small amount to test for any adverse reactions.

4. Chamomile Tea for Bloating

Beneficial effects:

Chamomile tea is renowned for its calming properties, which can significantly alleviate bloating and digestive discomfort. It acts as a natural anti-inflammatory agent, soothing the gastrointestinal tract, and facilitating gas expulsion to reduce bloating.

Portions

1 serving

Preparation time

5 minutes

Cooking time

10 minutes

Ingredients:

- 1 tablespoon of dried chamomile flowers or 1 chamomile tea bag

- 8 ounces of boiling water

- Honey or lemon (optional, for taste)

Instructions:

1. Boil 8 ounces of water in a kettle or pot.

2. Place the dried chamomile flowers or tea bag in a mug.

3. Pour the boiling water over the chamomile, ensuring it's fully submerged.

4. Cover the mug with a lid or a small plate and let it steep for 5 to 10 minutes. This allows the chamomile to fully infuse the water, extracting its beneficial properties.

5. Remove the cover and the chamomile flowers or tea bag from the mug.

6. If desired, add honey or a squeeze of lemon to taste.

7. Stir gently to combine if you've added honey or lemon.

8. Enjoy the tea while it's still warm for the best therapeutic effects.

Variations:

- For additional digestive support, add a slice of fresh ginger or a pinch of fennel seeds to the tea while it steeps.

- Mint leaves can also be added for their soothing properties and to enhance the flavor.

Storage tips:

- Chamomile tea is best enjoyed fresh, but if you need to store it, keep it in a thermos to retain its warmth and beneficial properties for up to a few hours.

Tips for allergens:

- Individuals with allergies to plants in the daisy family should avoid chamomile, as it may cause allergic reactions. As an alternative, peppermint tea can be used for similar digestive soothing effects without the risk of such allergies.

Scientific references:

- Srivastava, J. K., Shankar, E., & Gupta, S. (2010). Chamomile: A herbal medicine of the past with a bright future (Review). Molecular Medicine Reports, 3(6), 895–901. This study highlights chamomile's anti-inflammatory, anti-bacterial, and relaxant properties, supporting its use in treating digestive issues like bloating.

5. Caraway Seed Tincture

Beneficial effects: Caraway Seed Tincture is known for its ability to soothe digestive issues such as indigestion, bloating, and nausea. Its carminative properties help in reducing gas and spasms in the intestines, making it an excellent remedy for those looking to alleviate discomfort naturally.

Ingredients:

- 1/4 cup dried caraway seeds
- 1 cup vodka or any 40% alcohol

Instructions: 1. Place the dried caraway seeds in a clean, dry jar.

2. Pour the vodka over the seeds, ensuring they are completely submerged.

3. Seal the jar tightly and shake it to mix the contents.

4. Store the jar in a cool, dark place for 4 to 6 weeks. Shake the jar every few days to agitate the seeds.

5. After the infusion period, strain the tincture through a cheesecloth or fine mesh strainer into another clean, dry jar. Press or squeeze the seeds to extract as much liquid as possible.

6. Label the jar with the date and contents.

7. Your Caraway Seed Tincture is ready to use.

Dosage: Take 1-2 teaspoons of the tincture diluted in water or tea, up to three times a day, especially before meals or whenever experiencing digestive discomfort.

Storage tips: Store the tincture in a cool, dark place. It can last for up to 5 years if stored properly.

Tips for allergens: If you're allergic to caraway or other plants in the Apiaceae family, such as fennel or celery, it's best to avoid this tincture. Always consult with a healthcare provider before starting any new herbal remedy, especially if you have allergies or are pregnant or breastfeeding.

Variations: For a non-alcoholic version, glycerin can be used instead of vodka, though the extraction process may differ slightly and shelf life may be shorter.

Scientific references: Studies have shown that caraway seeds contain several essential oils and compounds that contribute to their medicinal properties, including carvone and limonene, which have been linked to digestive health benefits (Journal of Ethnopharmacology, 2019).

6. Lemon Balm Tea

Beneficial effects: Lemon Balm Tea is renowned for its calming effects, which can help alleviate stress, anxiety, and insomnia. It also offers digestive benefits, easing indigestion, bloating, and nausea. The natural compounds in lemon balm, such as rosmarinic acid, contribute to its soothing properties, making it a gentle remedy for both mind and body.

Ingredients:
- 1 tablespoon of dried lemon balm leaves or 1/4 cup of fresh lemon balm leaves
- 8 ounces of boiling water
- Honey or lemon (optional, to taste)

Instructions:

1. If using fresh lemon balm leaves, gently crush them with your hands to release the essential oils.

2. Place the lemon balm leaves in a tea infuser or directly in a cup.

3. Pour boiling water over the leaves and cover the cup with a lid or a small plate to trap the steam.

4. Let the tea steep for 5 to 10 minutes, depending on your desired strength.

5. Remove the tea infuser or strain the tea to remove the leaves.

6. Add honey or lemon to taste, if desired.

7. Enjoy the tea warm, ideally in a quiet, comfortable setting to enhance its calming effects.

Variations:

For a cooling summer beverage, allow the tea to cool to room temperature, then refrigerate for 1-2 hours. Serve over ice with a sprig of fresh mint or a slice of lemon for an extra refreshing twist.

Storage tips:

Dried lemon balm leaves should be stored in an airtight container in a cool, dark place to preserve their potency. Fresh lemon balm leaves can be kept in the refrigerator, wrapped in a damp paper towel and placed in a plastic bag, for up to a week.

Tips for allergens:

Those with allergies to plants in the mint family should proceed with caution when trying lemon balm for the first time. As always, consult with a healthcare provider if you have any concerns about potential allergies or interactions with other medications.

7. Dandelion Root Decoction

Beneficial effects: Dandelion root decoction is a potent herbal remedy known for its ability to support liver function, improve digestion, and reduce bloating and water retention. Its diuretic properties help flush toxins out of the body, making it an excellent choice for those seeking natural relief from indigestion, bloating, and nausea.

Ingredients:

- 1 tablespoon of dried dandelion root

- 1 cup of water

Instructions:

1. Bring 1 cup of water to a boil in a small saucepan.

2. Add 1 tablespoon of dried dandelion root to the boiling water.

3. Reduce the heat and simmer for about 10 minutes. This process extracts the beneficial compounds from the dandelion root.

4. Remove from heat and let it steep for an additional 10 minutes.

5. Strain the decoction into a cup, removing the dandelion root pieces.

6. Your dandelion root decoction is now ready to be enjoyed. It can be consumed 2-3 times daily, especially before meals to aid digestion.

Variations:

- For a sweeter taste, add a teaspoon of honey or maple syrup.

- Combine with ginger or peppermint in the decoction process to enhance its digestive benefits.

Storage tips:

- The dandelion root decoction is best consumed fresh but can be stored in the refrigerator for up to 48 hours. Ensure it is stored in a clean, airtight container.

Tips for allergens:

- Individuals with allergies to dandelion or other related plants should avoid this remedy.

Always consult with a healthcare provider before starting any new herbal treatment, especially if you have existing health conditions or are taking medications.

8. Licorice Root Tea

Beneficial effects:

Licorice root tea is known for its soothing properties that can help alleviate indigestion, bloating, and nausea. It also supports the health of the digestive system by enhancing mucous membrane protection in the stomach and intestines.

Portions

1 serving

Preparation time

5 minutes

Cooking time

10 minutes

Ingredients:

- 1 teaspoon of dried licorice root

- 8 ounces of boiling water

- Honey or lemon (optional, for taste)

Instructions

1. Place the dried licorice root in a tea infuser or tea bag.

2. Pour 8 ounces of boiling water over the licorice root.

3. Allow the tea to steep for 10 minutes. The longer it steeps, the stronger the flavor will be.

4. Remove the tea infuser or tea bag from the water.

5. If desired, add honey or a slice of lemon to taste.

6. Enjoy your licorice root tea warm.

Variations:

- For a cooler beverage, allow the tea to cool to room temperature, then refrigerate for 1-2 hours and serve over ice.

- Combine with ginger tea for an extra digestive health boost.

Storage tips:

Store dried licorice root in a cool, dry place away from direct sunlight to preserve its potency and flavor.

Tips for allergens:

Individuals with hypertension should consult with a healthcare provider before consuming licorice root tea, as it can affect blood pressure levels.

Scientific references:

- "The effect of licorice root on postoperative sore throat and cough after tracheal intubation." This study supports the anti-inflammatory properties of licorice root, which can soothe the digestive tract.

- "Deglycyrrhizinated licorice for peptic ulcer disease in adults." This review highlights the benefits of licorice root in protecting the mucous membranes of the stomach and intestines, which can help alleviate symptoms of indigestion and bloating.

9. Apple Cider Vinegar Drink

Beneficial effects:

Apple Cider Vinegar Drink is renowned for its potential to soothe indigestion, alleviate bloating, and mitigate nausea. Its acetic acid content can help improve digestion by increasing stomach acid, which in turn aids in breaking down food more efficiently. Additionally, it possesses natural antibacterial properties, which can combat nausea-causing bacteria. This remedy harnesses the simplicity of natural ingredients to offer relief from common digestive discomforts.

Ingredients:

- 1 tablespoon of organic apple cider vinegar (with "the mother" for extra benefits)
- 1 cup of warm water
- 1 teaspoon of raw honey (optional, for taste)
- A pinch of ground ginger (optional, for enhanced nausea relief)

Instructions:

1. Measure 1 tablespoon of organic apple cider vinegar.

2. Warm 1 cup of water to a comfortable drinking temperature. Avoid boiling water to preserve the beneficial enzymes in apple cider vinegar.

3. Combine the apple cider vinegar with the warm water in a mug or glass.

4. If desired, add 1 teaspoon of raw honey to the mixture. Stir well until the honey is fully dissolved.

5. For additional nausea relief, add a pinch of ground ginger to the concoction and mix thoroughly.

6. Consume the drink slowly. It's best taken before meals to aid digestion or at the first sign of indigestion or nausea.

Variations: For a refreshing twist, add a few slices of fresh apple or a squeeze of lemon juice to the drink.

- If you're experiencing severe bloating, a teaspoon of baking soda mixed into the drink can provide immediate relief by neutralizing stomach acid.

Storage tips:

This drink is best prepared fresh, but if you wish to prepare it in advance, store it in an airtight container in the refrigerator for up to 24 hours. Shake well before consuming if ingredients have settled or separated.

Tips for allergens:

If you're sensitive to honey, you can substitute it with maple syrup or simply omit the sweetener altogether. For those with a histamine intolerance, be cautious with apple cider vinegar as it may exacerbate symptoms in some individuals.

Scientific references:

- "Journal of Food Science," which discusses the antimicrobial properties of vinegar.

- "Digestive Diseases and Sciences," featuring a study on the effects of ginger on nausea and vomiting.

- A review in "The American Journal of Clinical Nutrition" highlights the potential health benefits of apple cider vinegar, including its impact on digestion and blood sugar regulation.

10. Turmeric and Ginger Smoothie

Beneficial effects:

This Turmeric and Ginger Smoothie is a powerhouse of anti-inflammatory and digestive benefits. Turmeric, with its active compound curcumin, offers potent anti-inflammatory properties that can help reduce bloating and indigestion. Ginger, known for its gastrointestinal relief, can soothe nausea and promote smooth digestion. Together, these ingredients create a smoothie that not only tastes great but also supports your digestive health and overall well-being.

Portions:

Serves 2

Preparation time:

10 minutes

Ingredients:

- 1 cup unsweetened almond milk
- 1 ripe banana, sliced and frozen
- 1/2 teaspoon ground turmeric
- 1/2 teaspoon grated fresh ginger
- 1/4 teaspoon ground cinnamon
- 1 tablespoon chia seeds
- 1 tablespoon honey, or to taste (optional for sweetness)
- Ice cubes (optional, for a thicker smoothie)

Instructions:

1. In a blender, combine the unsweetened almond milk, frozen banana slices, ground turmeric, grated fresh ginger, ground cinnamon, and chia seeds.

2. Blend on high until the mixture is smooth and creamy. If the smoothie is too thick, you can add a little more almond milk to reach your desired consistency.

3. Taste the smoothie and, if desired, add honey for sweetness. Blend again to incorporate the honey evenly.

4. If you prefer a colder, thicker smoothie, add a few ice cubes and blend until smooth.

5. Pour the smoothie into glasses and serve immediately.

Variations:

- For an extra protein boost, add a scoop of your favorite plant-based protein powder.

- Substitute almond milk with coconut milk for a creamier texture and tropical flavor.

- Add a handful of spinach or kale for added nutrients without significantly altering the taste.

Storage tips:

This smoothie is best enjoyed fresh, but if needed, it can be stored in the refrigerator for up to 24 hours. Be sure to stir or shake well before drinking if it has been sitting for a while.

Tips for allergens:

If you're allergic to almonds, any non-dairy milk alternative like coconut milk, oat milk, or soy milk can be used as a substitute for almond milk. Ensure to choose a brand that's safe for your specific allergies.

Scientific references:

- Hewlings, S.J., & Kalman, D.S. (2017). Curcumin: A Review of Its' Effects on Human Health. Foods, 6(10), 92. This study discusses the wide range of health benefits of curcumin, including its anti-inflammatory properties.

- Mashhadi, N.S., Ghiasvand, R., Askari, G., Hariri, M., Darvishi, L., & Mofid, M.R. (2013). Anti-oxidative and anti-inflammatory effects of ginger in health and physical activity: Review of current evidence. International Journal of Preventive Medicine, 4(Suppl 1), S36–S42. This review highlights ginger's effectiveness in relieving gastrointestinal irritation and its anti-inflammatory and antioxidant effects.

Recipes and Dosages

Crafting herbal remedies requires precision and understanding of the herbs' effects on the body. This section provides detailed recipes and dosages for creating safe, effective herbal treatments. Beginners will find the instructions straightforward, with clear explanations of each step and the reasons behind them. Emphasizing safety, each recipe includes guidelines to ensure that remedies are prepared correctly and effectively, minimizing the risk of adverse reactions.

11.   Ginger Tea for Digestive Relief

Objective: To soothe indigestion and nausea.

Preparation:

1. Boil 1 cup of water.

2. Peel and grate 1 teaspoon of fresh ginger root.

Materials:

- Fresh ginger root

- 1 cup of water

Tools:

- Teapot or saucepan

- Grater

- Strainer

Safety measures: Ensure ginger is fresh and free from mold.

Step-by-step instructions:

1. Add the grated ginger to boiling water.

2. Simmer for 10 minutes on low heat.

3. Strain the tea into a cup.

4. Allow to cool slightly before drinking.

Dosage: Drink 1 cup as needed for digestive discomfort, not exceeding 3 cups per day.

12.   Lavender Oil Sleep Aid

Objective: To promote relaxation and improve sleep quality.

Preparation:

1. Gather materials.

2. Ensure the workspace is clean.

Materials:

- 2 tablespoons of carrier oil (e.g., coconut or almond oil)

- 10 drops of lavender essential oil

Tools:

- Mixing bowl

- Small bottle or jar for storage

Safety measures: Perform a patch test on the skin to check for allergic reactions.

Step-by-step instructions:

1. Mix the lavender essential oil with the carrier oil in the bowl.

2. Transfer the mixture to the storage bottle.

3. Seal and label the bottle.

Dosage: Apply a small amount to the temples or wrists before bedtime. Use nightly as needed.

13. Chamomile Tea for Relaxation

Objective: To reduce stress and promote a sense of calm.

Preparation:

1. Boil 1 cup of water.

2. Measure 2 teaspoons of dried chamomile flowers.

Materials:

- Dried chamomile flowers

- 1 cup of water

Tools:

- Teapot or saucepan

- Measuring spoons

- Strainer

Safety measures: Ensure chamomile is free from contaminants.

Step-by-step instructions:

1. Add chamomile flowers to boiling water.

2. Cover and steep for 5 minutes.

3. Strain into a cup and let it cool slightly.

Dosage: Drink 1 cup in the evening to relax before bedtime. Do not exceed 2 cups per day.

14. Peppermint Oil Headache Relief

Objective: To alleviate headache symptoms.

Preparation:

1. Ensure all materials are ready and workspace is clean.

Materials:

- 2 tablespoons of carrier oil (e.g., jojoba or grapeseed oil)

- 4 drops of peppermint essential oil

Tools:

- Mixing bowl

- Small bottle or roller for application

Safety measures: Conduct a patch test to avoid skin irritation.

Step-by-step instructions:

1. Combine the peppermint oil with the carrier oil in the mixing bowl.

2. Transfer the blend to the application bottle.

3. Seal and label the bottle.

Dosage: Apply a small amount to the forehead and temples when experiencing headache symptoms. Use as needed, not exceeding 4 times per day.

15. Echinacea Tincture for Immune Support

Objective: To boost the immune system.

Preparation:

1. Gather dried Echinacea.

2. Measure 1 cup of high-proof alcohol.

Materials:

- 1 cup of dried Echinacea

- 2 cups of high-proof alcohol (e.g., vodka)

Tools:

- Glass jar with a tight-fitting lid

- Strainer or cheesecloth

- Funnel

- Dark-colored dropper bottles for storage

Safety measures: Use food-grade alcohol and ensure workspace is clean.

Step-by-step instructions:

1. Place Echinacea in the glass jar.

2. Cover with alcohol, ensuring herbs are completely submerged.

3. Seal the jar and store in a cool, dark place for 4-6 weeks, shaking it daily.

4. After maceration, strain the tincture through cheesecloth into a clean bowl.

5. Using a funnel, transfer the liquid into dropper bottles.

6. Label the bottles with the date and contents.

Dosage: Take 1-2 ml up to three times daily at the first sign of immune distress. Continue for up to two weeks.

These recipes and dosages serve as a foundation for beginners to explore the benefits of herbal remedies. Always consult with a healthcare professional before starting any new herbal regimen, especially if you have existing health conditions or are taking medications.

Respiratory health is a critical aspect of overall well-being, especially in a world where environmental factors, stress, and lifestyle choices can negatively impact lung function and breathing. Herbal remedies offer a natural way to support and enhance respiratory health, providing relief from symptoms associated with conditions like colds, coughs, and asthma. These remedies harness the power of plants to soothe irritation, reduce inflammation, and promote healing within the respiratory system.

16. Elderberry Syrup for Colds

Objective: To boost the immune system and alleviate cold symptoms.

Preparation:

1. Gather all materials.

Materials:

- 1 cup fresh or dried elderberries
- 4 cups water
- 1 cup raw honey
- A pot for boiling
- Strainer or cheesecloth
- Glass bottle or jar for storage

Safety measures: Ensure all utensils are clean to avoid contamination.

Step-by-step instructions:

1. Combine elderberries and water in a pot and bring to a boil.

2. Reduce heat and simmer until the liquid is reduced by half, approximately 45 minutes.

3. Strain the mixture through a cheesecloth or strainer into a bowl, pressing the berries to extract all the juice.

4. Allow the liquid to cool to room temperature, then stir in the honey.

5. Transfer the syrup to a glass bottle or jar and store in the refrigerator.

Dosage: Take 1 tablespoon daily for immune support or every 3-4 hours for cold relief.

17. Thyme and Honey Cough Syrup

Objective: To relieve cough and soothe the throat.

Preparation:

1. Prepare ingredients and tools.

Materials:

- 2 tablespoons dried thyme
- 1 cup water
- 1 cup honey
- Pot for boiling
- Strainer
- Glass jar for storage

Safety measures: Clean all tools thoroughly.

Step-by-step instructions:

1. Boil water and add thyme. Simmer for 10 minutes.

2. Strain the thyme leaves and mix the liquid with honey while still warm.

3. Store the syrup in a glass jar in the refrigerator.

Dosage: Take 1 teaspoon up to 4 times a day when experiencing a cough.

18.   Mullein Tea for Asthma

Objective: To reduce asthma symptoms and improve breathing.

Preparation:

1. Assemble materials.

Materials:

- 1-2 teaspoons dried mullein leaves

- 1 cup boiling water

- Teapot or cup

- Strainer

Safety measures: Ensure the mullein is free from contaminants.

Step-by-step instructions:

1. Place mullein leaves in a teapot or cup.

2. Pour boiling water over the leaves and steep for 10-15 minutes.

3. Strain and drink the tea.

Dosage: Consume 1-2 cups daily to support respiratory health.

19.   Eucalyptus Steam Inhalation

Objective: To clear congestion and ease breathing.

Preparation:

1. Prepare materials and set up a comfortable area for inhalation.

Materials:

- 3-5 drops eucalyptus essential oil

- Bowl of boiling water

- Towel

Safety measures: Be cautious with hot water to avoid burns. Use eucalyptus oil with care, especially around children and pets.

Step-by-step instructions:

1. Add eucalyptus oil to a bowl of boiling water.

2. Lean over the bowl and cover your head and the bowl with a towel to trap the steam.

3. Inhale deeply for 5-10 minutes.

Dosage: Perform once or twice daily, especially when experiencing congestion or respiratory discomfort.

20.   Garlic and Honey Elixir

Objective: To support immune function and combat respiratory infections.

Preparation:

1. Collect ingredients and a clean jar.

Materials:

- 1 cup raw honey

- 10-12 cloves of garlic, peeled and finely minced

- Jar with a lid

Safety measures: Ensure garlic is fresh and honey is of good quality.

Step-by-step instructions:

1. Mix minced garlic with honey in the jar until fully combined.

2. Seal the jar and let it sit for 3-7 days in a cool, dark place, mixing once daily.

3. After a week, strain if desired.

Dosage: Take 1 teaspoon on an empty stomach daily for immune support or every few hours when fighting a cold or respiratory infection.

These herbal remedies provide a natural approach to respiratory health, offering relief from symptoms while supporting the body's healing processes. Always consult with a healthcare professional before starting any new herbal treatment, especially if you have existing health conditions or are taking medications.

21. Elderberry Syrup for Colds

Beneficial effects:

Elderberry syrup is celebrated for its immune-boosting properties and ability to shorten the duration and severity of colds. Rich in antioxidants and vitamins, elderberry can help to fight inflammation and protect against viruses and bacteria.

Portions:

Makes approximately 2 cups

Preparation time:

10 minutes

Cooking time:

45 minutes

Ingredients:

- 3/4 cup dried elderberries
- 3 cups of water
- 1 teaspoon ground cinnamon
- 1/2 teaspoon ground cloves
- 1/2 teaspoon ground ginger
- 1 cup raw honey

Instructions:

1. Combine the dried elderberries, water, cinnamon, cloves, and ginger in a medium saucepan.

2. Bring the mixture to a boil, then reduce the heat and simmer, covered, for about 45 minutes or until the liquid has reduced by half.

3. Remove from heat and let the mixture cool to room temperature.

4. Mash the berries carefully using a spoon or potato masher.

5. Strain the mixture through a fine mesh strainer or cheesecloth into a large bowl, pressing on the berries to extract as much liquid as possible.

6. Discard the elderberries and let the liquid cool to lukewarm.

7. Once lukewarm, add the raw honey to the elderberry liquid and stir until well combined.

8. Transfer the syrup to a clean, sterilized glass jar or bottle.

Variations:

- For an extra immune boost, add a tablespoon of echinacea tincture to the finished syrup.

- If you prefer a vegan version, substitute honey with maple syrup or agave nectar, though keep in mind this will alter the flavor slightly.

Storage tips:

Store the elderberry syrup in the refrigerator. It will keep for up to two months. For longer storage, you can freeze the syrup in an ice cube tray and then transfer the cubes to a freezer bag for easy dosing.

Tips for allergens:

If you have allergies to berries, it's best to consult with a healthcare provider before taking elderberry syrup. For those allergic to honey, using a non-honey sweetener is a suitable alternative.

Scientific references:

- A study published in the "Journal of International Medical Research" found that when elderberry syrup was used within the first 48 hours of the onset of flu symptoms, it shortened the duration of the flu with symptoms being relieved on an average of four days earlier.

- Research in "Phytochemistry" identifies the flavonoids in elderberries as the primary active components, contributing to their antioxidant properties.

22.   Thyme and Honey Cough Syrup

Beneficial effects:

Thyme and Honey Cough Syrup is a time-honored remedy that harnesses the antiseptic and antimicrobial properties of thyme, combined with the soothing, anti-inflammatory benefits of honey, to provide relief for coughs, sore throats, and minor respiratory irritations. Thyme helps in loosening mucus, making it easier to cough up, while honey coats and soothes the throat, reducing cough severity and improving sleep quality.

Ingredients:

- 2 tablespoons of fresh thyme leaves or 1 tablespoon of dried thyme
- 1 cup of water
- 1 cup of honey

Instructions:

1. Bring the water to a boil in a small saucepan.

2. Add the thyme leaves to the boiling water and simmer for about 5 minutes.

3. Strain the thyme leaves from the water and pour the thyme-infused water into a heat-resistant measuring cup.

4. If necessary, add more water to the thyme infusion to make one cup.

5. Pour the thyme-infused water back into the saucepan and add the honey.

6. Heat the mixture over low heat, stirring constantly until the honey is fully dissolved and the mixture is well combined. Do not allow it to boil to preserve the beneficial properties of the honey.

7. Remove from heat and let the syrup cool.

8. Once cooled, pour the syrup into a clean, airtight glass jar.

Storage tips:

Store the Thyme and Honey Cough Syrup in the refrigerator for up to 3 months. Ensure the jar is tightly sealed to maintain freshness and prevent contamination.

Tips for allergens:

For those with allergies to honey, a suitable alternative is agave syrup or maple syrup, though it's important to note that the soothing effects might vary. Individuals with a known allergy to thyme or other herbs in the Lamiaceae family should avoid this remedy.

Variations:

- For an extra antimicrobial kick, add a tablespoon of freshly squeezed lemon juice to the mixture after removing it from heat.

- Incorporate a slice of ginger during the simmering process to enhance the syrup's anti-inflammatory properties.

23. Mullein Tea for Asthma

Beneficial effects:

Mullein tea is celebrated for its soothing properties on the respiratory system, making it an excellent choice for individuals dealing with asthma. Its anti-inflammatory and expectorant qualities help in reducing inflammation and easing the expulsion of mucus, providing relief from asthma symptoms such as wheezing, coughing, and breathlessness.

Ingredients:

- 1 to 2 teaspoons of dried mullein leaves
- 1 cup of boiling water
- Honey or lemon (optional, for taste)

Instructions:

1. Place the dried mullein leaves in a tea infuser or directly in a cup.

2. Pour 1 cup of boiling water over the mullein leaves.

3. Cover the cup with a lid or a small plate and let it steep for 10 to 15 minutes. This allows the therapeutic properties of the mullein to be released into the water.

4. Remove the tea infuser or strain the tea to remove the leaves.

5. If desired, add honey or lemon to taste. This can enhance the flavor and add additional soothing effects for the throat.

6. Drink the tea while it's warm to maximize its benefits for asthma relief.

Variations:

- For added respiratory support, combine mullein with other herbs such as ginger or peppermint, which have their own beneficial effects on the respiratory system.

- To create a stronger infusion, use more leaves and allow the tea to steep for a longer period.

Storage tips:

- Store dried mullein leaves in an airtight container in a cool, dark place to maintain their potency.

- It's best to prepare mullein tea fresh for each use, but any leftover tea can be stored in the refrigerator for up to 24 hours. Reheat gently without boiling before drinking.

Tips for allergens:

- Mullein is generally well-tolerated, but as with any herbal remedy, it's important to start with a small amount to ensure you do not have an allergic reaction, especially if you have sensitivities to plants in the figwort family.

- If you're using honey as a sweetener, ensure it's suitable for your dietary needs, especially if you have allergies to bee products.

Scientific references:

- A study published in the "Journal of Ethnopharmacology" highlights the anti-inflammatory properties of mullein, supporting its use in treating respiratory conditions like asthma.

- Research in the "American Journal of Respiratory and Critical Care Medicine" discusses the benefits of herbal expectorants, including mullein, in managing symptoms of chronic respiratory diseases.

24. Eucalyptus Steam Inhalation

Beneficial effects:

Eucalyptus steam inhalation is a traditional remedy known for its ability to relieve symptoms of colds, coughs, and asthma. The eucalyptus plant contains compounds that have both anti-inflammatory and expectorant properties, helping to clear the nasal passages, reduce congestion, and soothe irritated respiratory tracts.

Ingredients:

- 3 to 5 drops of eucalyptus essential oil
- 1 large bowl of boiling water
- A towel large enough to cover your head and the bowl

Instructions:

1. Carefully pour boiling water into the bowl.
2. Add 3 to 5 drops of eucalyptus essential oil to the hot water.
3. Lean over the bowl, and drape the towel over your head and the bowl, creating a tent that traps the steam.
4. Close your eyes to avoid irritation, and inhale the steam deeply for 5 to 10 minutes. You should start to feel your nasal passages opening and a soothing sensation in your throat.
5. Repeat up to 2 times a day as needed, especially before bed to help alleviate nighttime symptoms.

Variations:

- For additional relief, you can add a drop of peppermint oil or tea tree oil, which also have antimicrobial and decongestant properties.
- If you have sensitive skin, be cautious as the essential oils can cause irritation. Start with fewer drops of oil and adjust as tolerated.

Storage tips:

Eucalyptus essential oil should be stored in a cool, dark place away from direct sunlight to maintain its potency.

Tips for allergens:

If you have allergies to eucalyptus or other essential oils, it's best to perform a patch test before using this remedy. Apply a diluted drop of the essential oil to your skin and wait for 24 hours to check for any adverse reactions.

Scientific references:

- Studies have shown that eucalyptus oil has antimicrobial effects against many bacteria, viruses, and fungi, and it can help to alleviate symptoms of respiratory conditions. (Colds, Cough, and Asthma: The Effectiveness of Eucalyptus Steam Inhalation, Journal of Alternative and Complementary Medicine).
- Inhalation of eucalyptus essential oil was found to decrease subjective perceptions of nasal congestion and improve respiratory conditions in a clinical trial. (Eucalyptus Oil Inhalation Improves Respiratory Conditions:

A Controlled Clinical Trial, Respiratory Medicine Journal).

25. Garlic and Honey Elixir

Beneficial effects:

Garlic and Honey Elixir is a time-honored remedy known for its powerful combination to combat colds, coughs, and even asthma. Garlic has natural antibacterial and antiviral properties that help fight infections from the common cold or flu. Honey, on the other hand, acts as a natural cough suppressant and soothes sore throats, making this elixir a potent ally during cold and flu season.

Ingredients:

- 1 cup of raw, organic honey
- 10 cloves of garlic, peeled and finely minced

Instructions

1. In a small bowl, combine the minced garlic with the raw honey. Stir the mixture until the garlic is fully immersed in the honey.

2. Transfer the garlic and honey mixture to a jar with a tight-fitting lid.

3. Store the jar in a cool, dark place for 3 to 7 days to allow the garlic to infuse into the honey. Each day, gently stir the mixture or turn the jar upside down to ensure the garlic is well coated.

4. After a week, strain the garlic from the honey and store the infused honey in a clean jar. Keep the jar sealed and stored in a cool, dark place.

Dosage: For colds and coughs: Take 1 teaspoon of the Garlic and Honey Elixir every 2-3 hours as needed.

For asthma: Take 1 teaspoon of the elixir in the morning and another at night.

Variations:

- Add a teaspoon of ginger juice or a pinch of cayenne pepper to the mixture to enhance its decongestant properties.

- Incorporate a few sprigs of thyme or rosemary to the infusion for additional respiratory benefits.

Storage tips:

The Garlic and Honey Elixir can be stored in a cool, dark place for up to a month. For longer storage, keep it refrigerated where it can last for up to a year.

Tips for allergens:

Individuals who are allergic to garlic should avoid this remedy. As an alternative, a honey and ginger elixir can be used for similar benefits without garlic.

Scientific references

- "Journal of Nutrition Research" published a study highlighting the antimicrobial effects of garlic against common cold and flu viruses.

- "International Journal of Preventive Medicine" discusses honey's effectiveness as a natural cough suppressant and its role in soothing sore throats.

26. Elderflower Syrup

Beneficial effects:

Elderflower Syrup is renowned for its immune-boosting properties and its ability to alleviate symptoms of colds, flu, and allergies. Packed with antioxidants and anti-inflammatory compounds, elderflower can help reduce nasal congestion, soothe sore throats, and promote overall respiratory health.

Ingredients:

- 1 cup fresh elderflowers, gently rinsed and stems removed
- 2 cups water
- 2 cups sugar
- 1/4 cup lemon juice, freshly squeezed
- 2 teaspoons lemon zest

Instructions:

1. In a medium saucepan, bring the water and sugar to a boil, stirring until the sugar has completely dissolved.

2. Lower the heat, and add the elderflowers, lemon juice, and lemon zest to the saucepan.

3. Simmer the mixture on low heat for 20 minutes, allowing the flavors to infuse.

4. Remove the saucepan from heat and let the mixture cool to room temperature.

5. Once cooled, strain the syrup through a fine mesh sieve or cheesecloth into a clean bottle or jar, pressing on the elderflowers to extract as much liquid as possible.

6. Seal the bottle or jar and store in the refrigerator.

Variations:

- For a sugar-free version, substitute sugar with an equal amount of honey or your preferred sweetener, adjusting to taste.
- Add a sprig of mint or a few slices of ginger during the simmering process for an additional flavor profile.

Storage tips:

The Elderflower Syrup can be stored in the refrigerator for up to 2 weeks. For extended storage, the syrup can be frozen in ice cube trays and then transferred to a freezer bag, keeping it fresh for several months.

Tips for allergens:

Individuals with allergies to flowers should proceed with caution and may want to consult with a healthcare provider before consuming. For those avoiding citrus due to allergies, omit the lemon juice and zest and substitute with a dash of apple cider vinegar for a similar tangy effect.

27. Lavender Honey Syrup

Beneficial effects:

Lavender Honey Syrup combines the soothing properties of lavender, known for its ability to reduce anxiety, stress, and promote sleep, with the natural antibacterial and anti-inflammatory benefits of honey. This syrup is perfect for calming the mind before bedtime, alleviating sore throats, and providing a gentle immune boost.

Ingredients:

- 1 cup of raw, organic honey
- 2 tablespoons of dried lavender flowers
- 1 cup of water

Instructions:

1. Bring the water to a boil in a small saucepan.

2. Add the dried lavender flowers to the boiling water and reduce the heat. Simmer for about 15 minutes to create a strong lavender infusion.

3. Strain the lavender flowers from the water, squeezing out as much liquid as possible, and discard the flowers.

4. Return the lavender-infused water to the saucepan and add the honey.

5. Warm the mixture over low heat, stirring constantly, until the honey is completely dissolved into the lavender water. Do not boil to preserve the beneficial properties of the honey.

6. Remove from heat and allow the syrup to cool.

7. Once cooled, pour the syrup into a clean, sterilized glass bottle or jar.

Variations:

- For added respiratory benefits, especially during cold and flu season, add a teaspoon of fresh grated ginger or a few drops of eucalyptus oil to the mixture while simmering.
- If you prefer a thicker syrup, reduce the amount of water to 1/2 cup for a more concentrated infusion.

Storage tips:

Store your Lavender Honey Syrup in the refrigerator for up to 1 month. Ensure the container is tightly sealed to maintain freshness and prevent contamination.

Tips for allergens:

Individuals with allergies to pollen or bee products should proceed with caution when using honey-based remedies. As an alternative, agave syrup can be used in place of honey for those with allergies or dietary restrictions.

Scientific references:

- A study published in the "Journal of Medical Microbiology" found that honey has significant antibacterial properties, making it effective in treating and preventing infections.
- Research in "Phytotherapy Research" highlights lavender's anxiolytic (anxiety-reducing) effects, supporting its use in promoting relaxation and improving sleep quality.

---

28. Rosehip Tea

Beneficial effects:

Rosehip Tea is celebrated for its high vitamin C content, antioxidants, and anti-inflammatory properties. It can help boost the immune system, fight inflammation, and improve skin health. Its diuretic properties also support kidney health and can help in flushing toxins from the body.

Ingredients:

- 1 tablespoon of dried rosehips

- 8 ounces of boiling water

- Honey or lemon (optional, for taste)

Instructions:

1. Place the dried rosehips in a tea infuser or directly in a cup.

2. Pour 8 ounces of boiling water over the rosehips.

3. Cover and let steep for 10 to 15 minutes. The longer it steeps, the more potent the tea will be.

4. Remove the tea infuser or strain the tea to remove the rosehips.

5. If desired, add honey or lemon to taste.

6. Enjoy the tea warm, ideally in the morning to kickstart your day or in the evening to wind down.

Variations:

- For a fruity twist, add a slice of orange or apple during the steeping process.

- Combine with hibiscus flowers for an additional antioxidant boost and a vibrant color.

Storage tips: Store dried rosehips in a cool, dark place in an airtight container to maintain their potency and freshness. Prepared rosehip tea can be refrigerated in a sealed container and enjoyed cold, but it's best consumed within 24 hours for optimal benefits.

Tips for allergens:

Those with specific plant allergies should consult with a healthcare provider before consuming rosehip tea. For individuals sensitive to citrus or acidic foods, starting with a weaker infusion and gradually increasing the strength can help minimize any potential adverse reactions.

29. Hibiscus Tea

Beneficial effects:

Hibiscus tea is celebrated for its high vitamin C content and antioxidants, which can help boost the immune system, lower blood pressure, and reduce inflammation. Its diuretic properties also assist in flushing toxins from the body, promoting overall kidney health.

Ingredients:

- 2 tablespoons of dried hibiscus flowers

- 4 cups of water

- Honey or natural sweetener to taste (optional)

- A slice of lemon or lime for garnish (optional)

Instructions:

1. Bring water to a boil in a large pot.

2. Once boiling, remove from heat and add the dried hibiscus flowers.

3. Cover the pot and let the tea steep for 15-20 minutes, depending on your desired strength.

4. Strain the tea into a pitcher or individual cups, discarding the hibiscus flowers.

5. If desired, sweeten with honey or your choice of natural sweetener.

6. Garnish with a slice of lemon or lime to enhance flavor.

7. Serve the tea hot, or chill in the refrigerator to serve cold.

Variations:

- For a spicy twist, add a cinnamon stick or a few cloves while the tea is steeping.
- Mix hibiscus tea with sparkling water for a refreshing, fizzy drink.
- Combine hibiscus tea with green tea for added antioxidants and a unique flavor blend.

Storage tips:

- Hibiscus tea can be stored in the refrigerator for up to one week. Ensure it's kept in a sealed pitcher or bottle to maintain freshness.
- Dried hibiscus flowers should be stored in a cool, dry place in an airtight container to preserve their color and flavor.

Tips for allergens:

- Hibiscus tea is naturally caffeine-free and suitable for those who are sensitive to caffeine.
- If you're using honey as a sweetener, ensure it's pure and free from additives that could cause allergies.

---

30. Sage and Honey Syrup

Beneficial effects:

Sage and Honey Syrup combines the antimicrobial properties of sage with the soothing effects of honey, making it an excellent remedy for sore throats, coughs, and minor respiratory irritations. Sage has been traditionally used for its antiseptic and anti-inflammatory benefits, while honey acts as a natural cough suppressant.

Ingredients:

- 1 cup of water
- 1/4 cup fresh sage leaves or 2 tablespoons dried sage
- 1 cup of raw, organic honey

Instructions:

1. Bring the water to a boil in a small saucepan.
2. Add the sage leaves to the boiling water and reduce the heat. Simmer for about 10 minutes to allow the sage to infuse.
3. Remove from heat and let the mixture cool to room temperature.
4. Strain the sage leaves from the water, squeezing them to extract as much liquid as possible.
5. While the sage infusion is still warm (but not hot), stir in the honey until it's completely dissolved.
6. Transfer the syrup to a clean, airtight glass jar.

Variations:

- For additional respiratory support, add a teaspoon of fresh lemon juice or a pinch of cayenne pepper to the syrup after adding the honey.
- To enhance the syrup's soothing effects, incorporate a tablespoon of apple cider vinegar.

Storage tips:

Store the Sage and Honey Syrup in the refrigerator for up to a month. Ensure the jar is tightly sealed to maintain freshness and prevent contamination.

Tips for allergens:

Individuals with allergies to pollen or bee products should proceed with caution when using honey. A high-quality, pure maple syrup can be used as an alternative sweetener, though the texture and flavor of the syrup will differ.

31. Marshmallow Root Tea

Beneficial effects:

Marshmallow Root Tea is celebrated for its soothing effect on the digestive and respiratory systems. It contains mucilage, a gelatinous substance that coats and soothes the throat, stomach, and intestines, providing relief from irritation and inflammation. This makes it an excellent remedy for coughs, sore throats, indigestion, and acid reflux.

Ingredients:

- 2 tablespoons of dried marshmallow root
- 16 ounces (about 2 cups) of water
- Honey or lemon (optional, for taste)

Instructions:

1. Place the dried marshmallow root in a pot and add the water.

2. Cover the pot and bring to a boil, then reduce the heat and simmer for 15 to 20 minutes.

3. Remove from heat and let it steep for another 10 to 15 minutes with the lid on.

4. Strain the tea into a cup or mug, pressing on the marshmallow root to extract as much liquid as possible.

5. If desired, add honey or lemon to taste.

6. Enjoy the tea warm for the best soothing effects.

Variations:

- For additional respiratory support, add a pinch of ground ginger or cinnamon while simmering.

- Combine with peppermint tea to enhance the soothing effect on the digestive system.

Storage tips:

Dried marshmallow root should be stored in a cool, dark place in an airtight container to maintain its potency. The prepared tea can be refrigerated in a sealed container for up to 3 days. Gently reheat before consuming but do not boil, as this can reduce its effectiveness.

Tips for allergens:

If you are sensitive to any specific ingredients or have a history of allergies to other herbs, start with a small amount of marshmallow root tea to ensure no adverse reactions occur. Those with diabetes should be cautious when adding honey and consult with a healthcare provider, as marshmallow root can affect blood sugar levels.

Scientific references:

- Studies have shown that marshmallow root can act as an effective mucilage, forming a protective layer on the mucous membranes and providing relief from irritation (Journal of Ethnopharmacology, 2011).

- Research indicates that marshmallow root may help in treating coughs and colds by soothing the throat and reducing irritation (Phytotherapy Research, 2010).

32. Nettle Leaf Tea

Beneficial effects:

Nettle Leaf Tea is renowned for its natural anti-inflammatory properties, making it an excellent remedy for alleviating symptoms of allergies, such as hay fever, and providing relief from joint pain. It is also a diuretic, which can help flush toxins from the body, and is rich in nutrients, including vitamins A, C, and K, as well as several B vitamins, minerals like calcium, iron, magnesium, phosphorus, potassium, and sodium, fatty acids, amino acids, polyphenols, and pigments – many of which have antioxidant properties.

Ingredients:

- 1 tablespoon of dried nettle leaves
- 1 cup of boiling water
- Honey or lemon (optional, for taste)

Instructions

1. Place the dried nettle leaves in a tea infuser or directly into a mug.
2. Pour 1 cup of boiling water over the nettle leaves.
3. Cover the mug with a lid or a small plate to allow the tea to steep, keeping the steam and essential oils contained.
4. Let the tea steep for 10 to 15 minutes, depending on how strong you prefer your tea.
5. Remove the tea infuser or strain the tea to remove the loose leaves.
6. Add honey or lemon to taste, if desired.
7. Enjoy the tea warm, ideally in a calm environment to enhance its soothing effects.

Variations:

- To enhance the flavor and add additional health benefits, consider adding a slice of ginger or a dash of cinnamon.

- For a refreshing summer drink, allow the tea to cool and serve it over ice with a slice of lemon.

Storage tips:

- Dried nettle leaves should be stored in an airtight container in a cool, dark place to preserve their potency.
- Once brewed, nettle leaf tea can be kept in the refrigerator for up to 2 days. Ensure it's stored in a sealed container to maintain its freshness and prevent absorption of other flavors or odors.

Tips for allergens:

- While nettle leaf tea is generally safe for most people, those with allergies to plants in the Urticaceae family should proceed with caution.
- If you're using honey as a sweetener, ensure it's suitable for your dietary needs, especially if you have allergies to bee products.

33. Oregano Tea

Beneficial effects:

Oregano Tea is celebrated for its potent antibacterial, antiviral, and anti-inflammatory properties. It can provide relief for respiratory issues, such as coughs and sore throats, and aid in digestion. The active compounds in oregano, particularly carvacrol and thymol, are responsible for its therapeutic effects.

Ingredients:

- 1 tablespoon of fresh oregano leaves or 1 teaspoon of dried oregano

- 1 cup of boiling water
- Honey or lemon (optional, for taste)

Instructions

1. Place the oregano leaves in a tea infuser or directly in a cup.

2. Pour 1 cup of boiling water over the oregano leaves.

3. Cover the cup with a lid or a small plate and let it steep for 5 to 10 minutes.

4. Remove the tea infuser or strain the tea to remove the leaves.

5. If desired, add honey or lemon to taste, which can enhance the flavor and add additional health benefits.

6. Enjoy the tea warm, ideally 2-3 times a day, especially during cold and flu season or when experiencing digestive discomfort.

Variations:

- For a stronger immune boost, add a slice of ginger or a pinch of cayenne pepper while steeping.

- Combine with peppermint or echinacea tea for added respiratory support.

Storage tips:

- Store dried oregano in an airtight container in a cool, dark place to maintain its potency.

- It's best to prepare oregano tea fresh, but if necessary, you can store it in the refrigerator for up to 24 hours. Reheat gently without boiling before consuming.

Tips for allergens:

- Individuals with allergies to the Lamiaceae family (mint family), which includes oregano, should proceed with caution and may want to consult with a healthcare provider before trying oregano tea.

- If using honey as a sweetener, ensure it's suitable for your dietary needs, especially if you have allergies to bee products.

34.   Yarrow Tea

Beneficial effects:

Yarrow Tea is known for its ability to promote digestion, reduce fever, and support wound healing. Its natural anti-inflammatory properties make it an excellent remedy for soothing cold symptoms and providing relief from menstrual cramps.

Ingredients:

- 1 to 2 teaspoons of dried yarrow flowers
- 1 cup of boiling water

Instructions:

1. Place the dried yarrow flowers in a tea infuser or directly into a cup.

2. Pour 1 cup of boiling water over the yarrow flowers.

3. Cover the cup and let it steep for 5 to 10 minutes. The longer it steeps, the stronger the tea will be.

4. Remove the tea infuser or strain the tea to remove the flowers.

5. The tea can be enjoyed as is or sweetened with honey or lemon to taste.

Variations:

- For additional respiratory support, mix yarrow with peppermint or elderflower. This combination enhances the tea's soothing effects on the respiratory system.

- To aid in digestion, combine yarrow with ginger or fennel seeds, which can help to reduce bloating and improve digestive health.

Storage tips:

Store dried yarrow flowers in an airtight container in a cool, dark place to maintain their potency and extend their shelf life.

Tips for allergens:

Individuals with allergies to plants in the Asteraceae family, such as daisies, chrysanthemums, or ragweed, should proceed with caution when trying yarrow tea for the first time. Start with a small amount to test for any adverse reactions.

Scientific references:

- A study published in the "Journal of Ethnopharmacology" highlights yarrow's anti-inflammatory and antispasmodic properties, supporting its use in traditional medicine for pain relief and healing.
- Research in the "Journal of Agricultural and Food Chemistry" has identified several antioxidant compounds in yarrow, suggesting its potential benefits in protecting against oxidative stress.

35. Calendula Tea

Beneficial effects:

Calendula tea is known for its soothing, anti-inflammatory properties, making it an excellent choice for healing skin irritations, soothing sore throats, and enhancing digestive health. Its antiseptic qualities also assist in healing minor wounds and infections from the inside out.

Ingredients:

- 1 tablespoon of dried calendula flowers
- 8 ounces of boiling water
- Honey or lemon (optional, for taste)

Instructions:

1. Place the dried calendula flowers in a tea infuser or directly in a mug.
2. Pour 8 ounces of boiling water over the calendula flowers.
3. Cover the mug with a lid or a small plate and allow it to steep for 10 to 15 minutes. The longer it steeps, the more potent the infusion will be.
4. Remove the tea infuser or strain the tea to remove the flowers.
5. Optionally, add honey or lemon to taste.
6. Enjoy the tea warm, ideally 2-3 times a day, especially if using it for therapeutic purposes.

Variations:

- For a more complex flavor or additional health benefits, blend calendula with other herbs such as chamomile for relaxation, peppermint for digestion, or ginger for its anti-inflammatory properties.
- To make a cooling, soothing drink for irritated skin or sunburn, allow the tea to cool completely and apply it to the affected area with a clean cloth.

Storage tips:

Store dried calendula flowers in a cool, dark place in an airtight container to maintain their potency. Prepared calendula tea can be refrigerated in a sealed container for up to 48 hours. Reheat gently without boiling or enjoy cold.

Tips for allergens:

Individuals with allergies to plants in the Asteraceae family, such as daisies, chrysanthemums, or ragweed, should proceed with caution when trying calendula for the first time. Always consult with a healthcare provider if unsure about potential allergies.

Skin and Hair Care

Skin and hair care are integral to overall health and well-being, reflecting internal physiological states and environmental interactions. Embracing herbal remedies offers a gentle yet effective approach to nurturing skin and hair, leveraging nature's bounty to nourish, repair, and protect. This section delves into crafting herbal solutions tailored for skin and hair care needs, focusing on natural ingredients that are easily accessible and simple to prepare.

Objective: To create herbal remedies that support skin health and promote healthy hair using natural, plant-based ingredients.

Preparation:

1. Identify skin or hair concerns (e.g., dry skin, acne, dandruff, hair loss).

2. Choose herbs known for their beneficial properties related to your specific needs.

Materials:

- Herbs such as aloe vera, chamomile, rosemary, nettle, and lavender
- Carrier oils (e.g., coconut, jojoba, almond)
- Essential oils for added benefits and aroma
- Beeswax for salves and balms
- Distilled water or hydrosols
- Glass jars, bottles, and containers for storage

Tools:

- Double boiler for melting and blending ingredients
- Blender or mortar and pestle for creating herb powders
- Fine mesh strainer or cheesecloth for filtering
- Funnel for transferring liquids
- Measuring cups and spoons

Safety measures:

- Conduct patch tests for new ingredients to check for skin sensitivities.
- Sterilize all tools and containers before use to prevent contamination.
- Label all products with ingredients and date of creation for safety and reference.

Step-by-step instructions:

1. **Herbal Oil Infusion for Hair and Scalp**:

- Gently heat 1 cup of carrier oil with 2 tablespoons of dried rosemary and nettle leaves in a double boiler for 2 hours on low heat, ensuring the oil does not overheat.
- Strain the oil using a cheesecloth into a clean jar.
- Apply to the scalp and hair as a pre-shampoo treatment or leave-in conditioner.

2. **Chamomile and Lavender Face Toner**:

- Boil 1 cup of distilled water and pour over 1 tablespoon each of dried chamomile and lavender flowers.

- Allow to steep until cool, then strain and transfer to a glass bottle.

- Use a cotton ball to apply to the face after cleansing for soothing hydration.

3. **Aloe Vera and Tea Tree Acne Gel**:

- Extract gel from an aloe vera leaf and blend with 10 drops of tea tree essential oil.

- Store in a glass jar and apply a small amount to blemishes as a spot treatment.

4. **Rosemary Hair Rinse for Shine and Growth**:

- Simmer 2 tablespoons of dried rosemary leaves in 2 cups of water for 15 minutes.

- Allow to cool, then strain. Use as a final rinse after shampooing to stimulate hair growth and add shine.

5. **Calendula Salve for Dry Skin**:

- Melt 2 tablespoons of beeswax in a double boiler, then add 1 cup of calendula-infused oil.

- Stir well and pour into small tins or jars to solidify.

- Apply to dry or irritated skin areas as needed.

Cost estimate: Varies, but starting with small batches helps minimize costs, with most ingredients available for under $50 total.

Time estimate: Preparation time ranges from 30 minutes to 2 hours, not including infusion or cooling periods.

Safety tips:

- Keep water out of homemade products to extend shelf life and prevent bacterial growth.

- Store products in a cool, dark place to preserve the integrity of the oils and herbs.

Troubleshooting:

- If a salve is too hard, remelt and add more oil. If too soft, add more beeswax.

- If an infusion doesn't have the desired strength, allow more time or add more herbs initially.

Maintenance: Check stored products regularly for any changes in smell, texture, or color, which could indicate spoilage.

Difficulty rating: ★☆☆☆☆ to ★★☆☆☆, depending on the complexity of the recipe.

Variations:

- Customize herbal blends based on personal preferences or specific skin and hair needs.

- Experiment with different carrier and essential oils for varied therapeutic effects and fragrances.

By incorporating these herbal remedies into your skin and hair care routines, you embrace a holistic approach to beauty, grounded in the healing power of plants. These natural solutions offer a harmonious balance between efficacy and gentleness, catering to the body's needs without harsh chemicals or synthetic additives.

36.   Tea Tree Oil Acne Treatment

Beneficial effects:

Tea Tree Oil Acne Treatment harnesses the powerful antiseptic and anti-inflammatory properties of tea tree oil to combat acne. This natural remedy helps to cleanse the skin, reduce inflammation, and fight the bacteria that cause acne, leading to clearer, healthier skin over time.

Ingredients:

- 2 to 3 drops of tea tree essential oil
- 1 tablespoon of aloe vera gel
- 1 teaspoon of distilled water (optional, for sensitive skin)

Instructions:

1. In a small bowl, mix the tea tree oil with the aloe vera gel. If you have sensitive skin, dilute the mixture with distilled water to lessen the concentration.

2. Cleanse your face thoroughly with a gentle cleanser and pat dry.

3. Apply the tea tree oil and aloe vera mixture directly to the affected areas using a cotton swab or your fingertips. Be sure to avoid the area around the eyes.

4. Leave the treatment on your skin for about 20-30 minutes or overnight, depending on your skin's sensitivity.

5. Rinse off the treatment with warm water and pat your face dry with a clean towel.

6. Apply a non-comedogenic moisturizer to keep your skin hydrated.

Variations:

- For an all-over facial treatment, you can increase the quantities and mix 5 drops of tea tree oil with 2 tablespoons of aloe vera gel and spread evenly over your entire face.
- Add a drop of lavender oil to the mixture for additional anti-inflammatory benefits and to enhance the scent.

Storage tips:

The tea tree oil and aloe vera mixture should be prepared fresh for each application to ensure potency and prevent contamination. Store tea tree oil and aloe vera gel in a cool, dark place to maintain their efficacy.

Tips for allergens:

If you have sensitive skin or are prone to allergies, perform a patch test on a small area of your skin before applying the treatment to your face. If irritation occurs, dilute the mixture with more aloe vera gel or water, or discontinue use.

37. Aloe Vera Gel for Eczema

Beneficial effects:

Aloe Vera Gel is widely recognized for its soothing, moisturizing, and healing properties, making it an ideal remedy for eczema. This natural treatment helps to reduce skin inflammation, alleviate itching, and promote the healing of dry, cracked skin commonly associated with eczema.

Ingredients:

- 1 large Aloe Vera leaf

- 1 teaspoon of Vitamin E oil (optional, for added moisture)

Instructions:

1. Carefully slice the Aloe Vera leaf lengthwise to open it.

2. Use a spoon to scoop out the clear, gel-like substance inside the leaf.

3. Transfer the Aloe Vera gel to a blender and blend for a minute to ensure a smooth consistency.

4. If using, add the Vitamin E oil to the blended Aloe Vera gel and mix thoroughly.

5. Pour the mixture into a clean, airtight container.

Variations:

- For extra soothing effects, you can add a few drops of lavender or chamomile essential oil to the Aloe Vera gel. These oils are known for their calming properties and can help further reduce eczema-related inflammation and irritation.

- For a thicker consistency, mix the Aloe Vera gel with shea butter to create a more substantial barrier on the skin, which can be especially beneficial during dry, cold months.

Storage tips:

Store your Aloe Vera gel in the refrigerator for up to one week. For extended storage, freeze the gel in an ice cube tray and transfer the cubes to a freezer bag, keeping them frozen until needed. Thaw a cube at room temperature before use.

Tips for allergens:

If you have sensitive skin or are prone to allergies, patch test the Aloe Vera gel on a small area of your skin before applying it to larger areas affected by eczema. This is especially important when adding essential oils or Vitamin E oil, as these can sometimes cause irritation in sensitive individuals.

38. Rosemary and Lavender Hair Tonic

Beneficial effects:

Rosemary and Lavender Hair Tonic is a natural remedy designed to strengthen hair, stimulate growth, and reduce hair loss. Rosemary enhances circulation to the scalp, which can promote hair growth, while lavender oil is known for its ability to soothe the scalp and prevent dandruff. Together, they create a potent tonic that not only nourishes the hair but also imbues it with a pleasant fragrance.

Ingredients:

- 1/4 cup dried rosemary leaves

- 1/4 cup dried lavender flowers

- 2 cups water

- 1 tablespoon apple cider vinegar (optional, for shine)

Instructions:

1. Bring the water to a boil in a medium saucepan.

2. Add the dried rosemary leaves and lavender flowers to the boiling water.

3. Reduce the heat and simmer for 20-30 minutes, allowing the herbs to infuse their oils into the water.

4. Remove from heat and let the mixture cool to room temperature.

5. Strain the mixture, discarding the herbs, and pour the liquid into a clean bottle or jar. If using, add the apple cider vinegar to the mixture.

6. To use, apply the tonic to the scalp and hair after shampooing. Massage gently for a few minutes, then rinse with cool water or leave it in for additional benefit.

Variations:

- For an extra moisturizing effect, add a teaspoon of jojoba oil or argan oil to the tonic before applying.

- If you have dry hair, consider adding a few drops of glycerin to the mixture to help lock in moisture.

Storage tips:

Store the hair tonic in a cool, dark place. If refrigerated, it can last for up to 2 weeks. Ensure the bottle or jar is tightly sealed to preserve its potency.

Tips for allergens: Individuals with sensitivities to rosemary or lavender should perform a patch test on the skin before applying the tonic to the scalp. If irritation occurs, discontinue use immediately.

39. Burdock Root Salve for Eczema

Beneficial effects:

Burdock Root Salve is renowned for its potent anti-inflammatory and antibacterial properties, making it an excellent natural remedy for eczema. By soothing the skin, reducing redness, and promoting healing, this salve can offer relief from the itching and discomfort associated with eczema flare-ups.

Ingredients:

- 1/4 cup dried burdock root
- 1/2 cup coconut oil
- 1/4 cup shea butter
- 2 tablespoons beeswax
- 10 drops lavender essential oil (optional for additional soothing effects)

Instructions:

1. Combine the dried burdock root and coconut oil in a double boiler. Heat gently for 30 minutes to allow the burdock root to infuse into the oil.

2. Strain the mixture through a cheesecloth or fine mesh strainer to remove the burdock root. Discard the root and return the infused oil to the double boiler.

3. Add shea butter and beeswax to the infused oil. Heat until the beeswax and shea butter have melted completely and are well combined with the oil.

4. Remove from heat and let the mixture cool slightly.

5. If using, add the lavender essential oil to the mixture and stir well.

6. Pour the mixture into a clean jar or tin and allow it to solidify.

7. Once solidified, cover with a lid and label the container with the contents and date.

Variations:

- For extra moisturizing properties, add a tablespoon of almond oil or vitamin E oil to the mixture.

- If you prefer a vegan option, substitute beeswax with an equal amount of candelilla wax.

Storage tips:

Store the salve in a cool, dry place. If stored properly, the salve can last for up to a year. Avoid exposing it to direct sunlight or heat, as this can cause the salve to melt.

Tips for allergens: If you have sensitivities to any of the ingredients, especially essential oils, you can omit them from the recipe or substitute them with another oil that suits your skin better. Always perform a patch test on a small area of your skin before applying the salve extensively, especially if you have sensitive skin.

40.　*Green Tea and Honey Face Mask*
Beneficial effects:

The Green Tea and Honey Face Mask combines the antioxidant properties of green tea with the soothing and antibacterial benefits of honey, making it an excellent natural remedy for acne, eczema, and even

helping to prevent hair loss by improving scalp health. Green tea is rich in catechins, which help to reduce inflammation and fight bacteria, while honey is a natural humectant that moisturizes the skin, promoting a healthy, glowing complexion.

Ingredients:

- 1 tablespoon of green tea leaves or 1 green tea bag
- 1 cup of boiling water
- 2 tablespoons of raw, organic honey

Instructions:

1. Steep the green tea leaves or tea bag in boiling water for 3 to 5 minutes.

2. Remove the tea leaves or bag and allow the tea to cool to room temperature.

3. Mix 2 tablespoons of the brewed green tea with 2 tablespoons of raw, organic honey in a bowl until you achieve a paste-like consistency.

4. Apply the mask evenly over your clean face, avoiding the eye area.

5. Leave the mask on for 15-20 minutes.

6. Rinse off the mask with lukewarm water and pat your face dry with a soft towel.

Variations:

- For added exfoliation, mix in a teaspoon of fine sugar to the mask before applying.

- To enhance the mask's soothing effects, add a tablespoon of aloe vera gel.

Storage tips:

It's best to prepare the Green Tea and Honey Face Mask fresh for each use. However, any leftover brewed green tea can be stored in the refrigerator for up to 2 days and used as a toner or for making another batch of the mask.

Tips for allergens:

Individuals with allergies to pollen or bee products should proceed with caution when using honey. A patch test on a small area of the skin is recommended to ensure no allergic reaction occurs. For those allergic to green tea or other ingredients, consider substituting with chamomile tea, which also has soothing properties.

41. Neem Oil for Acne

Beneficial effects:

Neem oil is renowned for its potent anti-inflammatory, antimicrobial, and antiseptic properties, making it an effective natural remedy for acne. It helps to reduce redness and inflammation, combat bacterial infections that can cause acne, and promote clearer, healthier skin.

Ingredients:

- 1 tablespoon of organic, cold-pressed neem oil
- 2 tablespoons of aloe vera gel (to soothe and hydrate the skin)
- 3 to 4 drops of tea tree oil (optional, for added antimicrobial benefits)

Instructions:

1. In a clean bowl, mix 1 tablespoon of neem oil with 2 tablespoons of aloe vera gel.

2. If using, add 3 to 4 drops of tea tree oil to the mixture for enhanced antimicrobial effects.

3. Stir the ingredients together until well combined.

4. Apply a small amount of the mixture directly to the affected areas using a cotton swab or clean fingertips.

5. Leave the treatment on for about 20 to 30 minutes or overnight for more severe cases.

6. Rinse off with lukewarm water and pat your skin dry with a clean towel.

7. For best results, use this remedy once daily, preferably at night, to reduce acne and improve skin health.

Variations:

- For sensitive skin, dilute the neem oil with a carrier oil like jojoba or sweet almond oil before mixing with aloe vera gel.

- Add a few drops of lavender oil to the mixture for its calming properties and to help reduce skin irritation.

Storage tips:

Store any leftover mixture in a small, airtight container in the refrigerator for up to one week. Ensure the container is clean and sterilized to prevent bacterial growth.

Tips for allergens:

- Always conduct a patch test on a small area of skin before applying the treatment to larger areas, especially if you have sensitive skin or are prone to allergic reactions.

- If you're allergic to neem, aloe vera, tea tree, or any other ingredient listed, avoid using this remedy. Consult with a healthcare provider for alternative treatments suitable for your skin type and condition.

42. Oatmeal Bath for Eczema

Beneficial effects:

An oatmeal bath is a gentle and effective remedy for soothing eczema. The natural properties of oatmeal help in moisturizing the skin, reducing inflammation, and alleviating the itchiness associated with eczema. Its antioxidant and anti-inflammatory compounds provide a protective barrier, aiding in skin healing.

Ingredients:

- 1 cup of colloidal oatmeal (finely ground oatmeal)
- Lukewarm water for a full bath

Instructions

1. Grind the oatmeal in a food processor or blender until it becomes a fine powder, ensuring it's colloidal to avoid any coarse bits that might not dissolve well in water.

2. Fill the bathtub with lukewarm water. Avoid hot water, as it can further irritate and dry out the skin.

3. Gradually sprinkle the colloidal oatmeal into the tub as it fills, stirring the water with your hand to ensure even distribution.

4. Once the bath is ready, soak in the oatmeal bath for 15 to 20 minutes. Use this time to relax and let the oatmeal's natural properties soothe the skin.

5. After soaking, gently pat the skin dry with a soft towel. Avoid rubbing the skin, as this can cause irritation.

6. Immediately apply a moisturizer to lock in hydration and protect the skin barrier.

Variations:

- For additional soothing effects, add a few drops of lavender or chamomile essential oil to the bath. These oils can help reduce stress and further soothe irritated skin.

- For a more moisturizing effect, mix in a tablespoon of coconut oil or almond oil with the colloidal oatmeal before adding it to the bath.

Storage tips:

- Store unused colloidal oatmeal in an airtight container in a cool, dry place to keep it fresh and ready for your next bath.

Tips for allergens:

- Ensure you're not allergic to oats. While rare, some individuals with eczema may have sensitivities to oats. Test on a small area of skin before taking a full bath.

- If adding essential oils, confirm you don't have sensitivities or allergies to them. Essential oils are potent, and a patch test is recommended before use.

43. Horsetail Hair Rinse

Beneficial effects:

Horsetail Hair Rinse leverages the high silica content found in horsetail herb, which is known for strengthening hair, enhancing hair growth, and improving scalp circulation. This natural remedy can help reduce hair loss, combat dandruff, and restore shine and texture to your hair, making it an excellent addition to your hair care routine.

Ingredients:

- 1/4 cup dried horsetail herb

- 4 cups of water

Instructions:

1. Bring the water to a boil in a large pot.

2. Add the dried horsetail herb to the boiling water.

3. Reduce the heat and let it simmer for 20 to 30 minutes. This process allows the water to become infused with the silica and other beneficial compounds from the horsetail.

4. After simmering, remove the pot from the heat and allow the mixture to cool to room temperature.

5. Strain the mixture, discarding the horsetail herb, and collect the infused water in a clean container.

6. To use, shampoo your hair as usual, then pour the horsetail hair rinse through your hair as a final rinse. Do not rinse out with water.

7. Repeat this treatment once or twice a week for best results.

Variations:

- For additional benefits, you can add a few drops of essential oils such as rosemary or lavender to the horsetail rinse. These oils can further stimulate hair growth and provide a pleasant scent.

- If dealing with an itchy or particularly flaky scalp, adding a tablespoon of apple cider vinegar to the rinse can help balance scalp pH and combat dandruff.

Storage tips:

The horsetail hair rinse can be stored in the refrigerator for up to one week. Ensure it's kept in a sealed container to maintain its potency. Shake well before each use as natural sediments may settle at the bottom.

Tips for allergens:

Individuals with sensitivities to herbal products should patch test the horsetail rinse on a small section of their skin before applying it to their scalp to ensure there is no adverse reaction.

44. Calendula Cream for Eczema

Beneficial effects:

Calendula cream is renowned for its anti-inflammatory and healing properties, making it an ideal remedy for soothing and treating eczema. Its natural compounds can help reduce itching, redness, and dryness associated with eczema flare-ups.

Ingredients:

- 1/4 cup calendula-infused oil
- 1/8 cup shea butter
- 1/8 cup coconut oil
- 1 tablespoon beeswax
- 10 drops lavender essential oil (optional for additional soothing effects)

Instructions:

1. In a double boiler, gently melt the shea butter, coconut oil, and beeswax together.

2. Once melted, remove from heat and stir in the calendula-infused oil.

3. Allow the mixture to cool slightly before adding the lavender essential oil, if using.

4. Pour the mixture into a clean, dry container and let it solidify. You can speed up this process by placing it in the refrigerator.

5. Once solidified, your calendula cream is ready to use. Apply a small amount to the affected area 2-3 times a day, or as needed.

Variations:

- For a vegan version, replace beeswax with an equal amount of candelilla wax.

- If coconut oil is too heavy for your skin, jojoba oil can be used as a lighter alternative.

Storage tips:

Store your calendula cream in a cool, dry place away from direct sunlight. If stored properly, it can last for up to 6 months. For longer shelf life, keep it refrigerated.

Tips for allergens:

- If you're sensitive to lavender or any other essential oils, you can omit them from the recipe.

- For those with nut allergies, ensure that the shea butter is processed in a facility free of nut contaminants or substitute it with mango butter.

45. Witch Hazel Toner for Acne

Beneficial effects:

Witch Hazel Toner for Acne leverages the astringent and anti-inflammatory properties of witch hazel to reduce acne and inflammation. It helps in tightening pores, soothing irritation, and promoting clearer skin.

Ingredients:

- 1/2 cup of witch hazel extract
- 1/4 cup of distilled water
- 10 drops of tea tree oil
- 5 drops of lavender essential oil

Instructions:

1. In a clean, sterilized bottle, combine the witch hazel extract and distilled water.

2. Add the tea tree oil and lavender essential oil to the mixture.

3. Close the bottle and shake well to ensure all the ingredients are thoroughly mixed.

4. To use, apply the toner gently to the face with a cotton pad, avoiding the eye area. Use morning and night after cleansing and before moisturizing.

Variations:

- For sensitive skin, reduce the amount of tea tree oil to 5 drops to minimize the risk of irritation.

- Add aloe vera gel for its soothing and hydrating properties, especially beneficial for inflamed or irritated skin.

Storage tips:

Store the toner in a cool, dark place. The shelf life is approximately 6 months. If the toner develops an off smell or color, it should be discarded.

Tips for allergens:

Individuals with sensitivity to tea tree or lavender oil should perform a patch test on a small area of skin before applying the toner to their face. Alternatively, these essential oils can be omitted or replaced with milder options like chamomile oil.

Topical Treatments and Masks

Creating natural topical treatments and masks offers a gentle yet effective way to care for your skin using the healing power of herbs. These remedies can soothe, nourish, and rejuvenate the skin, addressing issues such as dryness, acne, and signs of aging without the harsh chemicals found in many commercial products. Here, we'll explore how to make your own herbal face masks and treatments with ingredients that are likely already in your kitchen or garden, ensuring an accessible and holistic approach to skincare.

Objective: To craft natural and effective topical treatments and masks for various skin concerns using herbal ingredients.

Preparation:

1. Determine your skin type and any specific concerns you wish to address, such as acne, dryness, or sensitivity.

2. Select herbs and natural ingredients known for their skin-healing properties that match your skin's needs.

Materials:

- Base ingredients: honey, yogurt, or clay for mask bases
- Herbs: chamomile, calendula, green tea, lavender, rosemary
- Oils: jojoba, almond, coconut, or olive oil for their moisturizing properties
- Essential oils: tea tree, lavender, or rose for added benefits and fragrance
- Fresh ingredients: cucumber, avocado, or aloe vera for hydration and vitamins

Tools:

- Blender or mortar and pestle to grind herbs and mix ingredients
- Mixing bowl and spoon
- Measuring spoons and cups
- Strainer or cheesecloth for filtering herbal infusions

Safety measures:

- Conduct a patch test on your inner arm with each new ingredient to ensure no allergic reaction occurs.
- Ensure all tools and surfaces are clean to prevent contamination of your skincare products.

Step-by-step instructions:

1. Herbal Infused Honey Mask:

- Gently warm 2 tablespoons of honey without overheating.

- Mix in 1 teaspoon of finely ground chamomile and lavender flowers.

- Apply to clean, damp skin and leave on for 15-20 minutes before rinsing with warm water.

2. **Green Tea and Yogurt Soothing Mask**:

- Brew a strong cup of green tea and allow it to cool.

- Mix 1 tablespoon of plain yogurt with 1 teaspoon of cooled green tea and a teaspoon of honey.

- Apply to the face for 15-20 minutes, then rinse with cool water.

3. **Calendula and Clay Healing Mask**:

- Prepare a calendula infusion by steeping 2 tablespoons of calendula flowers in hot water for 15 minutes. Strain and cool.

- Mix 2 tablespoons of clay (bentonite or kaolin) with enough calendula infusion to form a paste.

- Apply to the face and let it dry for 10-15 minutes, then rinse with lukewarm water.

4. **Avocado and Olive Oil Moisture Mask**:

- Mash half an avocado and mix with 1 tablespoon of olive oil.

- Apply to clean, dry skin and leave on for 20 minutes. Rinse with warm water and pat dry.

5. **Cucumber and Aloe Vera Cooling Gel**:

- Blend half a cucumber with 2 tablespoons of aloe vera gel until smooth.

- Apply to the face for a cooling effect, especially after sun exposure. Rinse off after 10-15 minutes.

Cost estimate: Most ingredients can be found in your kitchen or garden, making each mask cost-effective, typically under $5 per application.

Time estimate: Preparation time is about 10-15 minutes, with an additional 15-20 minutes for application.

Safety tips:

- Always use fresh and organic ingredients to minimize the risk of pesticides or chemicals.

- Discard any leftover mask mixture, as these natural remedies do not contain preservatives and can spoil quickly.

Troubleshooting:

- If a mask is too runny, add more solid ingredients like clay or ground oats to thicken.

- If a mask is too thick, slowly mix in more liquid (water, herbal infusion, or oil) until the desired consistency is achieved.

Maintenance: Clean all tools and containers thoroughly after use to prevent the growth of bacteria.

Difficulty rating: ★☆☆☆☆. These recipes are designed to be simple and accessible, even for beginners.

Variations:

- Personalize your mask by adding different herbal infusions or essential oils based on your skin's needs.
- Experiment with seasonal fruits and vegetables for additional vitamins and antioxidants.

By incorporating these herbal treatments and masks into your skincare routine, you can enjoy the benefits of natural ingredients and the satisfaction of creating your own personalized products. These gentle remedies offer a holistic approach to skin health, allowing you to nurture your skin with the healing power of nature.

46. Turmeric and Black Pepper Paste

Beneficial effects:

Turmeric and Black Pepper Paste combines the powerful anti-inflammatory properties of curcumin, found in turmeric, with piperine from black pepper, enhancing the absorption and effectiveness of curcumin in the body. This paste can help reduce inflammation, pain, and improve overall health.

Ingredients:

- 1/2 cup of turmeric powder
- 1 cup of water (plus additional water if needed)
- 1 1/2 teaspoons of ground black pepper
- 1/4 cup of coconut oil, or olive oil

Instructions:

1. Combine the turmeric powder and water in a saucepan. Start with 1 cup of water, adding more if necessary, to form a paste.

2. Cook over medium-low heat, stirring constantly, until a thick paste forms, about 7-10 minutes.

3. Add the ground black pepper and coconut oil to the turmeric paste. Stir well to incorporate all the ingredients thoroughly.

4. Allow the mixture to cool.

5. Once cooled, transfer the paste to a glass jar with a tight-fitting lid.

Variations: For added benefits, include a teaspoon of ground cinnamon or ginger to the paste for their antioxidant properties.

- Substitute coconut oil with olive oil if preferred, as both offer health benefits and can aid in the absorption of turmeric.

Storage tips:

Store the turmeric and black pepper paste in the refrigerator for up to 2 weeks. Ensure the jar is tightly sealed to maintain freshness and potency.

Tips for allergens:

- If you are allergic to turmeric, black pepper, or coconut, please avoid this remedy.

- For those with a sensitivity to coconut oil, olive oil is an excellent alternative that does not compromise the effectiveness of the paste.

47. Willow Bark Tea

Beneficial effects:

Willow Bark Tea is known for its natural anti-inflammatory and pain-relieving properties, making it an effective remedy for reducing pain and inflammation associated with conditions like arthritis, headaches, and menstrual cramps. The active component, salicin, acts similarly to aspirin, providing relief without the harsh side effects of synthetic medications.

Ingredients:

- 2 teaspoons of dried willow bark
- 8 ounces of water

Instructions:

1. Bring 8 ounces of water to a boil in a small saucepan.

2. Add 2 teaspoons of dried willow bark to the boiling water.

3. Reduce the heat and simmer for 10 to 15 minutes. This allows the salicin in the willow bark to infuse into the water.

4. Remove from heat and let it steep for an additional 30 minutes.

. Strain the tea into a cup, discarding the willow bark.

6. Enjoy the tea warm. It can be consumed up to 2-3 times a day for pain relief.

Variations:

- For added flavor and additional anti-inflammatory benefits, consider adding a slice of ginger or a stick of cinnamon to the tea while it simmers.

- If the taste is too bitter, sweeten the tea with a teaspoon of honey or maple syrup.

Storage tips:

Prepare willow bark tea fresh for each use to ensure maximum potency and effectiveness. Dried willow bark should be stored in a cool, dry place, in an airtight container, away from direct sunlight.

Tips for allergens:

Individuals who are allergic to aspirin or other salicylates should avoid willow bark tea, as it contains similar compounds. Always consult with a healthcare provider before trying new herbal remedies, especially if you are pregnant, nursing, or taking other medications.

48. Ginger and Turmeric Compress

Beneficial effects:

The Ginger and Turmeric Compress offers a natural and effective way to alleviate pain and reduce inflammation. Ginger, with its potent anti-inflammatory properties, works in tandem with turmeric, which contains curcumin, a compound known for its ability to decrease swelling and pain. This remedy is particularly beneficial for those suffering from arthritis, muscle soreness, or injuries.

Ingredients:

- 1 tablespoon of freshly grated ginger
- 1 tablespoon of turmeric powder
- 1 cup of water
- A clean cloth or towel

Instructions:

1. Bring 1 cup of water to a boil in a small saucepan.

2. Add the freshly grated ginger and turmeric powder to the boiling water.

3. Reduce the heat and let the mixture simmer for 10 minutes.

4. Remove the saucepan from the heat and allow it to cool slightly, just enough so it can be applied to the skin without causing burns.

5. Soak the clean cloth or towel in the ginger and turmeric mixture, then wring out the excess liquid.

6. Apply the compress to the affected area for 15-20 minutes.

7. Repeat 2-3 times a day as needed for pain relief and to reduce inflammation.

Variations:

- For enhanced anti-inflammatory effects, add a teaspoon of crushed garlic to the simmering water. Garlic has additional anti-inflammatory and analgesic properties.

- If the smell of turmeric and ginger is too strong, add a few drops of lavender oil to the compress for its calming scent and additional anti-inflammatory benefits.

Storage tips:

The ginger and turmeric mixture can be stored in the refrigerator for up to 2 days. Warm slightly before soaking the cloth and applying as a compress.

Tips for allergens:

Individuals with allergies to ginger, turmeric, or latex (for the cloth) should perform a patch test on a small area of skin before applying the compress to larger areas. If irritation or allergic reaction occurs, discontinue use immediately.

---

49. Boswellia Serrata Capsules

Beneficial effects:

Boswellia Serrata Capsules are recognized for their potent anti-inflammatory properties, making them an effective natural remedy for managing pain and inflammation associated with conditions like arthritis, inflammatory bowel disease (IBD), and asthma. The active compounds in Boswellia, such as boswellic acids, have been shown to inhibit pro-inflammatory enzymes, providing relief from swelling and pain without the side effects commonly associated with synthetic drugs.

Ingredients:

- 450 mg of Boswellia Serrata extract (standardized to contain 65% boswellic acids)
- Vegetable capsule shells

Instructions:

1. If starting with Boswellia Serrata resin, grind the resin into a fine powder using a mortar and pestle or a coffee grinder.

2. Measure 450 mg of the Boswellia Serrata powder and carefully fill the empty vegetable capsule shells. Use a capsule filling machine for ease and accuracy, if available.

3. Close the capsules according to the manufacturer's instructions.

4. Label the container with the date and contents.

Dosage:

Take one capsule up to two times daily with water, preferably after meals, or as directed by a healthcare provider.

Variations:

- For enhanced joint support, Boswellia Serrata capsules can be combined with other natural anti-inflammatory supplements such as turmeric or ginger capsules.

- Individuals with more severe inflammation may consider a higher dosage, but only under the guidance of a healthcare professional.

Storage tips:

Store the capsules in a cool, dry place, away from direct sunlight. Ensure the container is tightly sealed to maintain potency.

Tips for allergens: Boswellia Serrata is generally well-tolerated; however, individuals with known sensitivities to herbal supplements should begin with a lower dose to assess tolerance.

- Ensure the vegetable capsule shells are free from allergens that may affect you, such as soy or gluten.

50.   Devil's Claw Root Tea

Beneficial effects:

Devil's Claw Root Tea is known for its anti-inflammatory and analgesic properties, making it an effective natural remedy for relieving pain and inflammation associated with conditions like arthritis, gout, and general muscle pain. It works by inhibiting pathways involved in inflammation, offering a natural alternative to over-the-counter pain medications.

Ingredients:

- 1 teaspoon of dried devil's claw root
- 1 cup of boiling water
- Honey or lemon to taste (optional)

Instructions:

1. Place the dried devil's claw root into a tea infuser or directly into a cup.

2. Pour 1 cup of boiling water over the devil's claw root.

3. Cover the cup and allow it to steep for 8 to 10 minutes. The longer it steeps, the stronger the tea will be.

4. Remove the tea infuser or strain the tea to remove the loose root pieces.

5. If desired, add honey or lemon to taste for flavor.

6. Drink the tea while warm, up to two times a day, to help reduce pain and inflammation.

Variations:

- For added anti-inflammatory benefits, mix in a half teaspoon of turmeric powder before steeping.

- Combine with ginger tea for an additional warming effect that can further soothe muscle and joint pain.

Storage tips:

Store dried devil's claw root in a cool, dry place away from direct sunlight to preserve its potency. Prepared devil's claw tea can be refrigerated in a sealed container for up to 2 days. Warm gently before consuming, but do not re-boil.

Tips for allergens:

Individuals with allergies to plants in the sesame family should proceed with caution when trying devil's claw for the first time. As always, consult with a healthcare provider before starting any new herbal remedy, especially if you are pregnant, breastfeeding, or taking medication.

51.   Arnica Salve

Beneficial effects:

Arnica Salve is widely recognized for its remarkable anti-inflammatory and pain-relieving properties. It is particularly effective in treating bruises, sprains, and muscle soreness, reducing swelling and accelerating the healing process. Its natural components make it a safe alternative for those looking to alleviate pain without the use of synthetic medications.

Ingredients:

- 1/2 cup arnica-infused oil
- 1/4 cup coconut oil
- 1/4 cup beeswax
- 10 drops of lavender essential oil (optional, for added anti-inflammatory and calming effects)

Instructions:

1. Combine the arnica-infused oil, coconut oil, and beeswax in a double boiler over medium heat.

2. Stir the mixture continuously until the beeswax is completely melted and the ingredients are well combined.

3. Remove from heat and allow the mixture to cool slightly.

4. If using, stir in the lavender essential oil.

5. Carefully pour the mixture into small tins or jars.

6. Allow the salve to cool and solidify completely before securing the lids.

Variations:

- For extra pain relief, add 5 drops of peppermint essential oil to the mixture for its cooling effect.

- If you prefer a vegan option, substitute beeswax with an equal amount of candelilla wax or soy wax.

Storage tips:

Store the arnica salve in a cool, dark place. If stored properly, the salve can last for up to a year. Avoid exposing it to direct sunlight or heat as it can cause the salve to melt.

Tips for allergens:

Individuals who are allergic to arnica, coconut, beeswax, or lavender should either omit these ingredients or substitute them with suitable alternatives. Always perform a patch test on a small area of your skin before applying the salve extensively, especially if you have sensitive skin or known allergies.

52. St. John's Wort Oil

Beneficial effects:

St. John's Wort Oil is renowned for its anti-inflammatory and analgesic properties, making it an excellent natural remedy for relieving pain and inflammation. It is particularly effective for nerve-related pain such as sciatica, arthritis discomfort, and muscular aches. The active compounds in St. John's Wort, such as hypericin, help to soothe the nervous system and reduce inflammation, providing relief from pain and promoting healing.

Ingredients:

- 1 cup of fresh St. John's Wort flowers
- 2 cups of olive oil or almond oil

Instructions:

1. Harvest St. John's Wort flowers when they are in full bloom, which is typically around mid-summer.

2. Gently wash the flowers to remove any dirt or insects, and let them dry completely to avoid moisture in the oil.

3. Place the dried flowers in a clean, dry jar, filling it to the top without compacting them.

4. Pour the olive oil or almond oil over the flowers until the jar is full, ensuring the flowers are completely submerged.

5. Seal the jar tightly and place it in a sunny spot for 4 to 6 weeks, shaking it gently every few days.

6. After the infusion period, strain the oil through a cheesecloth or fine mesh strainer into another clean, dry jar. Press or squeeze the flowers to extract as much oil as possible.

7. Label the jar with the date and contents.

Variations:

- For added pain-relieving properties, you can infuse the oil with other herbs such as lavender or chamomile.

- To make a stronger infusion, use a double boiler to gently heat the oil and flowers for 2 to 3 hours instead of sun-infusing.

Storage tips:

Store the St. John's Wort Oil in a cool, dark place. It can last for up to 1 year if stored properly. Ensure the jar is tightly sealed to maintain its potency.

Tips for allergens:

Individuals sensitive to St. John's Wort or the base oil used (olive or almond) should perform a patch test on a small area of skin before applying broadly. If irritation occurs, discontinue use immediately.

53. Cayenne Pepper Balm

Beneficial effects:

Cayenne Pepper Balm is an effective natural remedy for pain relief and reducing inflammation. The capsaicin in cayenne pepper helps to decrease the intensity of pain signals sent through the body. Additionally, its warming effect improves blood circulation to the affected area, aiding in the healing process.

Ingredients:

- 1/4 cup coconut oil
- 2 tablespoons grated beeswax
- 1 teaspoon cayenne pepper powder
- 1/2 teaspoon ginger powder
- 1/2 teaspoon turmeric powder
- 15 drops peppermint essential oil

Instructions:

1. In a double boiler, gently melt the coconut oil and beeswax together until completely liquid.

2. Carefully stir in the cayenne pepper, ginger, and turmeric powders until well combined.

3. Remove the mixture from heat and allow it to cool slightly before adding the peppermint essential oil. Stir thoroughly to ensure even distribution of the oil.

4. Pour the mixture into a small jar or tin and let it solidify at room temperature, or place in the refrigerator to speed up the process.

5. Once solidified, cover with a lid and label the container with the contents and date.

Variations:

- For a stronger balm, increase the amount of cayenne pepper powder gradually, testing on a small skin area first to ensure it's not too intense.

- Add a few drops of lavender essential oil for additional soothing effects and a pleasant scent.

Storage tips:

Store the Cayenne Pepper Balm in a cool, dark place. If stored properly, it can last for up to a year. Keep the lid tightly closed to maintain its potency.

Tips for allergens:

- Individuals with sensitive skin or allergies to any of the ingredients should perform a patch test on a small area of skin before applying the balm extensively.

- If you're allergic to coconut oil, it can be substituted with another carrier oil such as almond oil or olive oil.

- Those sensitive to peppermint or other essential oils can reduce the amount used or omit it entirely.

54. White Willow Bark Tincture

Beneficial effects:

White Willow Bark Tincture is known for its natural pain-relieving and anti-inflammatory properties, making it an effective remedy for headaches, arthritis, and other inflammatory conditions. The active compound in white willow bark, salicin, is similar to aspirin, which helps in reducing pain and inflammation.

Ingredients:

- 1/4 cup dried white willow bark
- 1 cup vodka or 40% alcohol

Instructions:

1. Place the dried white willow bark into a clean, dry jar.
2. Pour the vodka over the bark, ensuring that the bark is completely submerged.
3. Seal the jar tightly and label it with the date and contents.
4. Store the jar in a cool, dark place for 4 to 6 weeks, shaking it every few days to mix the contents.
5. After the infusion period, strain the tincture through a cheesecloth or fine mesh strainer into another clean, dry jar. Press or squeeze the soaked bark to extract as much liquid as possible.
6. Label the jar with the date and contents.

Variations:

- For a non-alcoholic version, glycerin can be substituted for vodka, though the extraction process may differ and the resulting tincture may have a shorter shelf life.

- To enhance the anti-inflammatory effects, consider adding turmeric or ginger to the tincture during the infusion process.

Storage tips:

Store the tincture in a cool, dark place. When stored properly, it can last for up to 5 years.

Tips for allergens:

Individuals with allergies to salicylates (such as aspirin) should avoid using white willow bark tincture. Always consult with a healthcare provider before starting any new herbal remedy, especially if you have allergies, are pregnant, breastfeeding, or taking medication.

55. Comfrey Poultice

Beneficial effects:

Comfrey Poultice is renowned for its remarkable healing properties, particularly when it comes to reducing pain and inflammation. The active compound allantoin promotes cell regeneration, speeding up the healing process of bruises, sprains, and even broken bones. Its anti-inflammatory properties also make it an excellent choice for alleviating joint pain and inflammation.

Ingredients:

- 1/4 cup of fresh comfrey leaves (or 2 tablespoons of dried comfrey leaves)
- Water (enough to form a paste)
- 1 clean cloth or gauze

Instructions:

1. If using fresh comfrey leaves, wash them thoroughly to remove any dirt. If using dried comfrey, skip to step 2.

2. Crush the comfrey leaves using a mortar and pestle or blend them in a food processor to form a paste. Add a little water if necessary to achieve the desired consistency.

3. Spread the comfrey paste evenly onto the center of the cloth or gauze.

4. Apply the poultice directly to the affected area, ensuring the paste is in contact with the skin.

5. Secure the poultice with a bandage or another piece of cloth to keep it in place.

6. Leave the poultice on for up to 4 hours for adults or 2 hours for children. For sensitive skin, check the area frequently and remove if any irritation occurs.

7. After removing, gently wash the area with warm water and pat dry.

Variations:

- For added anti-inflammatory effects, mix a teaspoon of turmeric powder into the paste before applying.

- To enhance the poultice's soothing properties, add a few drops of lavender essential oil to the paste.

Storage tips:

Fresh comfrey leaves should be used immediately or stored in the refrigerator for up to 24 hours. Dried comfrey leaves can be stored in an airtight container in a cool, dark place for up to a year.

Tips for allergens:

Individuals with sensitive skin or allergies to comfrey should perform a patch test on a small area of skin before applying the poultice widely. If irritation or allergic reaction occurs, discontinue use immediately.

56. White Willow Bark Tea

Beneficial effects:

White Willow Bark Tea is celebrated for its natural pain-relieving properties, making it an effective remedy for headaches, arthritis pain, and other forms of discomfort. The active ingredient, salicin, works similarly to aspirin by reducing inflammation and blocking pain signals. This herbal tea offers a gentle alternative to over-the-counter pain medications, providing relief without the harsh side effects.

Ingredients:

- 2 teaspoons of dried white willow bark
- 8 ounces of water

Instructions:

1. Bring 8 ounces of water to a boil in a small saucepan or kettle.

2. Place the dried white willow bark into a tea infuser or directly into the boiling water.

3. Reduce the heat and simmer for 10 to 15 minutes. This allows the salicin in the white willow bark to be released into the water.

4. Remove from heat and let the tea steep for an additional 5 to 10 minutes, depending on the desired strength.

5. Strain the tea into a cup if you've added the bark directly to the water.

6. Enjoy the tea warm, up to 2-3 times a day, for natural pain relief.

Variations: - For additional flavor and health benefits, add a slice of ginger or a cinnamon stick to the tea while it simmers.

- To enhance the anti-inflammatory effects, mix in a half teaspoon of turmeric powder before simmering.

Storage tips:

Store leftover dried white willow bark in an airtight container in a cool, dark place to maintain its potency. Prepared white willow bark tea can be refrigerated in a sealed container for up to 48 hours. Warm gently before consuming, but do not re-boil.

Tips for allergens:

Individuals with allergies to aspirin or other salicylates should avoid white willow bark tea, as it contains similar compounds. Always consult with a healthcare provider before trying new herbal remedies, especially if you are pregnant, breastfeeding, or taking medication.

57. Turmeric and Black Pepper Paste

Beneficial effects:

Turmeric and Black Pepper Paste is a potent anti-inflammatory and antioxidant remedy, ideal for reducing pain and inflammation associated with conditions like arthritis, muscle soreness, and even enhancing overall well-being. The combination of curcumin in turmeric and piperine in black pepper increases the bioavailability of curcumin, making it more effective in its healing properties.

Ingredients:

- 1/2 cup of turmeric powder
- 1 cup of water (additional water may be needed)
- 1 1/2 teaspoons of ground black pepper
- 1/4 cup of coconut oil

Instructions:

1. Combine the turmeric powder and water in a saucepan, starting with 1 cup of water. Add more water as needed to form a smooth paste.

2. Heat the mixture over low to medium heat, stirring constantly, until it forms a thick paste. This process should take about 7-10 minutes.

3. Add the ground black pepper and coconut oil to the paste, continuing to stir until all the ingredients are fully integrated and the mixture is smooth.

4. Allow the paste to cool. Once cooled, transfer the paste into a glass jar with a tight-fitting lid.

Storage tips:

Keep the turmeric and black pepper paste in the refrigerator for up to 2 weeks. Ensure the jar is sealed properly to maintain freshness and prevent contamination.

Tips for allergens:

For individuals with coconut allergies, olive oil can be used as a substitute for coconut oil. Always ensure that you are not allergic to any of the ingredients used in the paste. Conduct a patch test if you are trying this remedy for the first time to ensure there is no adverse reaction.

58. Ginger and Turmeric Compress

Beneficial effects:

The Ginger and Turmeric Compress offers a natural and effective way to alleviate pain and reduce inflammation. Ginger, with its potent anti-inflammatory properties, works in tandem with turmeric, which contains curcumin, a compound known for its ability to decrease swelling and pain. This remedy is particularly beneficial for those suffering from arthritis, muscle soreness, or injuries.

Ingredients:

- 1 tablespoon of freshly grated ginger
- 1 tablespoon of turmeric powder
- 1 cup of water
- A clean cloth or towel

Instructions:

1. Bring 1 cup of water to a boil in a small saucepan.

2. Add the freshly grated ginger and turmeric powder to the boiling water.

3. Reduce the heat and let the mixture simmer for 10 minutes.

4. Remove the saucepan from the heat and allow it to cool slightly, just enough so it can be applied to the skin without causing burns.

5. Soak the clean cloth or towel in the ginger and turmeric mixture, then wring out the excess liquid.

6. Apply the compress to the affected area for 15-20 minutes.

7. Repeat 2-3 times a day as needed for pain relief and to reduce inflammation.

Variations:

- For enhanced anti-inflammatory effects, add a teaspoon of crushed garlic to the simmering water. Garlic has additional anti-inflammatory and analgesic properties.

- If the smell of turmeric and ginger is too strong, add a few drops of lavender oil to the compress for its calming scent and additional anti-inflammatory benefits.

Storage tips:

The ginger and turmeric mixture can be stored in the refrigerator for up to 2 days. Warm slightly before soaking the cloth and applying as a compress.

Tips for allergens:

Individuals with allergies to ginger, turmeric, or latex (for the cloth) should perform a patch test on a small area of skin before applying the compress to larger areas. If irritation or allergic reaction occurs, discontinue use immediately.

59. *Boswellia Serrata Capsules*

Beneficial effects:

Boswellia Serrata Capsules are known for their strong anti-inflammatory and pain-relieving properties. They can be particularly beneficial for individuals suffering from conditions like osteoarthritis, rheumatoid arthritis, and inflammatory bowel disease. By inhibiting pro-inflammatory enzymes and reducing leukotriene synthesis, Boswellia Serrata helps to decrease inflammation, alleviate pain, and improve mobility.

Ingredients:

- 450 mg of Boswellia Serrata extract (standardized to contain at least 65% boswellic acids)
- Vegetable capsule shells

Instructions:

1. If starting with Boswellia Serrata resin, first grind the resin into a fine powder using a coffee grinder or mortar and pestle.

2. Measure out 450 mg of the Boswellia Serrata powder.

3. Carefully fill the empty vegetable capsule shells with the measured powder. A capsule machine can be used for ease and accuracy.

4. Close the capsules as per the machine's or the manual method's instructions.

5. Label the container with the contents and the date of preparation.

Dosage

Take one capsule up to two times daily, preferably with meals, or as directed by a healthcare professional.

Variations:

- For individuals seeking additional anti-inflammatory support, consider combining Boswellia Serrata capsules with turmeric curcumin supplements, which can further enhance the anti-inflammatory effects due to the synergistic properties of curcumin and boswellic acids.

- Those looking for enhanced joint support may add glucosamine and chondroitin supplements to their regimen alongside Boswellia Serrata capsules.

Storage tips:

Store the capsules in a cool, dry place, away from direct sunlight. Ensure the container is tightly sealed to maintain the potency of the Boswellia Serrata extract.

Tips for allergens:

- Individuals with known allergies to herbal supplements should start with a lower dose to assess tolerance.

- Ensure the vegetable capsule shells are free from allergens that may affect you, such as soy or gluten. Always check the label of the capsule shells if you're purchasing them separately.

60. Devil's Claw Root Tea

Beneficial effects:

Devil's Claw Root Tea is celebrated for its anti-inflammatory and analgesic properties, making it a natural and effective remedy for relieving pain and inflammation. It is particularly beneficial for individuals suffering from arthritis, back pain, and other conditions characterized by inflammation and discomfort.

Ingredients:

- 1 teaspoon of dried devil's claw root
- 1 cup of boiling water
- Honey or lemon to taste (optional)

Instructions:

1. Place the dried devil's claw root into a tea infuser or directly into a cup.

2. Pour 1 cup of boiling water over the devil's claw root.

3. Cover the cup and allow it to steep for 8 to 10 minutes. The longer it steeps, the stronger the tea will be.

4. Remove the tea infuser or strain the tea to remove the loose root pieces.

5. If desired, add honey or lemon to taste for flavor.

6. Drink the tea while warm, up to two times a day, to help reduce pain and inflammation.

Variations:

- For added anti-inflammatory benefits, mix in a half teaspoon of turmeric powder before steeping.

- Combine with ginger tea for an additional warming effect that can further soothe muscle and joint pain.

Storage tips:

Store dried devil's claw root in a cool, dry place away from direct sunlight to preserve its potency. Prepared devil's claw tea can be refrigerated in a sealed container for up to 2 days. Warm gently before consuming, but do not re-boil.

Tips for allergens:

Individuals with allergies to plants in the sesame family should proceed with caution when trying devil's claw for the first time. As always, consult with a healthcare provider before starting any new herbal remedy, especially if you are pregnant, breastfeeding, or taking medication.

61. Arnica Salve

Beneficial effects:

Arnica Salve is widely praised for its anti-inflammatory and analgesic properties, offering a natural solution for relieving pain, reducing swelling, and accelerating the healing process of bruises, sprains, and muscle aches. Its active components, such as sesquiterpene lactones, help to mitigate inflammation and ease discomfort, making it an essential remedy for those seeking relief from various physical ailments without resorting to synthetic medications.

Ingredients:

- 1/2 cup arnica-infused oil
- 1/4 cup coconut oil
- 1/4 cup beeswax
- 10 drops of lavender essential oil (optional, for added soothing effects)

Instructions:

1. Combine the arnica-infused oil, coconut oil, and beeswax in a double boiler over medium heat.
2. Stir the mixture continuously until the beeswax is completely melted and the ingredients are well combined.
3. Remove from heat and allow the mixture to cool slightly.
4. If using, stir in the lavender essential oil.
5. Carefully pour the mixture into small tins or jars.
6. Allow the salve to cool and solidify completely before securing the lids.

Variations: - For those with sensitive skin, reduce the amount of arnica-infused oil to 1/4 cup and increase the coconut oil to 1/2 cup to dilute the potency.
- Add a few drops of peppermint essential oil for a cooling effect that can further aid in pain relief.

Storage tips:

Store the arnica salve in a cool, dark place. If stored properly, the salve can last for up to a year. Avoid exposing it to direct sunlight or heat as it can cause the salve to melt.

Tips for allergens:

- Individuals who are allergic to arnica, coconut, beeswax, or lavender should either omit these ingredients or substitute them with suitable alternatives.
- Always perform a patch test on a small area of your skin before applying the salve extensively, especially if you have sensitive skin or known allergies.

62. St. John's Wort Oil

Beneficial effects:

St. John's Wort Oil is celebrated for its remarkable ability to soothe nerve pain, reduce inflammation, and support the healing of wounds. Its active compounds, notably hypericin, have been studied for their effectiveness in treating mild to moderate depression, making this oil a versatile addition to natural health practices. When applied topically, it can offer relief from conditions like sciatica, muscular pain, and even help in the recovery of minor burns, bruises, and cuts by promoting skin regeneration.

Ingredients:

- 1 cup of fresh St. John's Wort flowers

- 2 cups of olive oil

Instructions:

1. Carefully pick the St. John's Wort flowers around midsummer, when they are in full bloom and the concentration of active compounds is highest.

2. Wash the flowers gently to remove any dirt or insects, and let them dry completely to avoid moisture in the oil, which could lead to spoilage.

3. Place the dried flowers in a clean, dry glass jar, filling it to about three-quarters full.

4. Pour the olive oil over the flowers until the jar is nearly full, ensuring that the flowers are completely submerged to prevent mold formation.

5. Close the jar tightly and place it in a sunny spot for about 4 to 6 weeks. This sun infusion method allows the oil to extract the active compounds from the flowers. Shake the jar gently every few days to mix the contents.

6. After the infusion period, strain the oil through a fine mesh strainer or cheesecloth into another clean, dry jar, pressing the flowers to extract as much oil as possible.

7. Label the jar with the date of production and contents.

Variations:

- For enhanced skin-healing properties, you can add a few drops of lavender or chamomile essential oil to the strained St. John's Wort Oil. These essential oils provide additional anti-inflammatory and soothing benefits.

- If olive oil is not preferred, almond oil can be used as an alternative carrier oil, offering a lighter texture suitable for facial application.

Storage tips:

Store the St. John's Wort Oil in a cool, dark place, such as a cupboard or a pantry, to preserve its potency. Properly stored, the oil can last for up to one year. Ensure the storage jar is tightly sealed to prevent oxidation.

Tips for allergens:

Individuals with known sensitivities to St. John's Wort should conduct a patch test before widespread application. Additionally, those sensitive to olive or almond oil can substitute with a more suitable carrier oil, like jojoba oil, which is generally well-tolerated by people with sensitive skin.

63. Cayenne Pepper Balm

Beneficial effects:

Cayenne Pepper Balm is a powerful natural remedy designed to alleviate pain and reduce inflammation. The capsaicin in cayenne pepper works by depleting the body's supply of substance P, a chemical component of nerve cells that transmits pain signals to the brain. This process provides relief from joint and muscle pain, nerve pain, and even headaches. Additionally, the warming effect of the balm improves circulation to the affected area, further aiding in the healing process.

Ingredients:

- 2 tablespoons cayenne pepper powder

- 1/2 cup coconut oil

- 1/4 cup beeswax pellets

- 10 drops of peppermint essential oil

- 5 drops of ginger essential oil

Instructions:

1. In a double boiler, gently melt the coconut oil and beeswax pellets together, stirring continuously until fully combined.

2. Carefully mix in the cayenne pepper powder, ensuring it's evenly distributed throughout the oil.

3. Remove the mixture from heat and let it cool slightly before adding the peppermint and ginger essential oils. Stir well to incorporate.

4. Pour the mixture into a clean, small jar or tin and allow it to cool and solidify completely.

5. Once solidified, secure the lid on the container.

Variations:

- For sensitive skin, reduce the amount of cayenne pepper powder to 1 tablespoon.

- To enhance the anti-inflammatory properties, add 5 drops of turmeric essential oil to the mixture.

Storage tips: Store the Cayenne Pepper Balm in a cool, dark place. If kept sealed and away from direct sunlight, the balm can last for up to a year.

Tips for allergens:

- Individuals with sensitive skin or allergies to any of the ingredients should perform a patch test on a small area of skin before using extensively.

- If allergic to coconut oil, substitute with an equal amount of almond oil or olive oil.

- Those sensitive to peppermint or ginger essential oils can reduce the amount used or omit them entirely.

64. White Willow Bark Tincture

Beneficial effects:

White Willow Bark Tincture serves as a natural pain reliever, offering a gentler alternative to synthetic aspirin. It's particularly effective for easing headaches, reducing arthritis discomfort, and soothing menstrual cramps. The active compound, salicin, found in white willow bark, is converted into salicylic acid in the body, which helps to diminish pain and inflammation.

Ingredients:

- 1/4 cup dried white willow bark

- 1 cup high-proof alcohol (such as vodka or grain alcohol)

Instructions:

1. Place the dried white willow bark into a clean, dry glass jar.

2. Pour the alcohol over the bark, ensuring that it is completely submerged.

3. Seal the jar tightly and label it with the date and contents.

4. Store the jar in a cool, dark place, shaking it daily, for 4 to 6 weeks.

5. After the infusion period, strain the tincture through a cheesecloth or fine mesh strainer into another clean, dry jar, squeezing or

pressing the bark to extract as much liquid as possible.

6. Label the final product with the date and store it in a cool, dark place.

Variations:

- For those sensitive to alcohol, a glycerin-based tincture can be made by substituting alcohol with vegetable glycerin and water (use a 3:1 ratio of glycerin to water).

- To enhance the anti-inflammatory effects, consider adding turmeric or ginger to the tincture during the infusion process.

Storage tips:

The tincture should be stored in a cool, dark place, away from direct sunlight. When stored properly, it can last for several years. Ensure the container is tightly sealed to prevent evaporation and degradation of the active compounds.

Tips for allergens:

Individuals with allergies or sensitivities to salicylates (the same compounds found in aspirin) should proceed with caution when using white willow bark tincture. Always start with a small dose to ensure no adverse reactions occur.

65. *Comfrey Poultice*

Beneficial effects:

Comfrey Poultice is recognized for its powerful healing properties, particularly in reducing pain and inflammation. It is highly effective for treating sprains, strains, bruises, and broken bones. Comfrey contains allantoin, a substance that speeds up the natural replacement of body cells, which contributes to the healing process. It is also known for its ability to alleviate pain, making it an excellent natural remedy for those seeking relief from discomfort caused by injuries or conditions like arthritis.

Ingredients:

- 1/4 cup of fresh comfrey leaves (or 2 tablespoons of dried comfrey leaves)
- Water (enough to form a paste)
- 1 clean cloth or gauze

Instructions:

1. Crush the comfrey leaves using a mortar and pestle or blend them in a food processor to form a paste. Add a little water if necessary to achieve the desired consistency.

2. Spread the comfrey paste evenly onto the center of the cloth or gauze.

3. Apply the poultice directly to the affected area, ensuring the paste is in contact with the skin.

4. Secure the poultice with a bandage or another piece of cloth to keep it in place.

5. Leave the poultice on for up to 4 hours for adults or 2 hours for children. For sensitive skin, check the area frequently and remove if any irritation occurs.

6. After removing, gently wash the area with warm water and pat dry.

Variations:

- For added anti-inflammatory effects, mix a teaspoon of turmeric powder into the paste before applying.

- To enhance the poultice's soothing properties, add a few drops of lavender essential oil to the paste.

Storage tips:

Fresh comfrey leaves should be used immediately or stored in the refrigerator for up to 24 hours. Dried comfrey leaves can be stored in an airtight container in a cool, dark place for up to a year.

Tips for allergens:

Individuals with sensitive skin or allergies to comfrey should perform a patch test on a small area of skin before applying the poultice widely. If irritation or allergic reaction occurs, discontinue use immediately.

66. *Turmeric Golden Milk*

Beneficial effects:

Turmeric Golden Milk is a traditional Ayurvedic drink known for its anti-inflammatory and antioxidant properties. It helps in reducing inflammation, boosting the immune system, and promoting overall wellness. The active ingredient in turmeric, curcumin, is enhanced by the presence of black pepper, increasing its bioavailability and effectiveness in the body.

Ingredients:

- 1 cup of milk (dairy or plant-based)
- 1 teaspoon of turmeric powder
- 1/2 teaspoon of ground cinnamon
- 1/4 teaspoon of ground ginger
- A pinch of ground black pepper
- 1 teaspoon of honey or maple syrup (optional, for sweetness)

Instructions:

1. In a small saucepan, combine milk, turmeric powder, ground cinnamon, ground ginger, and a pinch of ground black pepper.

2. Heat the mixture over medium heat, stirring constantly, until it is hot but not boiling.

3. Remove from heat and let it cool for a minute.

4. Stir in honey or maple syrup to taste, if using.

5. Pour the golden milk through a strainer into a mug to remove any large spice particles.

6. Enjoy warm.

Variations:

- For a vegan version, use almond milk, coconut milk, or any plant-based milk of your choice.

- Add a teaspoon of virgin coconut oil or ghee for added richness and to further enhance the absorption of turmeric.

- For an extra boost, add a small piece of fresh turmeric root (grated) in step 1, if available.

Storage tips:

It's best to enjoy Turmeric Golden Milk fresh. However, if you need to store it, keep it in a tightly sealed container in the refrigerator for up to 2 days. Reheat gently on the stove before drinking, as separation may occur in plant-based milks.

Tips for allergens:

- For those with dairy allergies or lactose intolerance, using plant-based milk ensures this remedy is both beneficial and enjoyable without discomfort.

- If you're allergic to any of the spices, they can be omitted or substituted with alternatives that don't cause you any adverse reactions.

67.   Boswellia Tea

Beneficial effects:

Boswellia Tea is known for its potent anti-inflammatory properties, making it an effective natural remedy for reducing inflammation and pain associated with conditions such as arthritis, inflammatory bowel disease, and asthma. The active compounds in Boswellia, known as boswellic acids, have been shown to inhibit the production of pro-inflammatory enzymes, offering relief without the side effects commonly associated with synthetic anti-inflammatory drugs.

Ingredients:

- 1 teaspoon of Boswellia serrata resin
- 1 cup of boiling water

Instructions:

1. Place the Boswellia serrata resin in a tea infuser or directly into a cup.

2. Pour 1 cup of boiling water over the resin.

3. Allow the tea to steep for 10 minutes. The longer it steeps, the stronger the infusion will be.

4. Remove the tea infuser or strain the tea to remove the resin pieces.

5. Enjoy the tea warm, ideally once in the morning and once in the evening for best results.

Variations:

- To enhance the flavor and add additional health benefits, consider adding a slice of ginger or a stick of cinnamon to the tea while it steeps.

- For those looking for a sweeter taste, a teaspoon of honey or maple syrup can be added after the tea has steeped.

Storage tips:

Store Boswellia serrata resin in a cool, dry place, away from direct sunlight, to maintain its potency. Prepared Boswellia Tea is best enjoyed fresh but can be stored in a refrigerator for up to 24 hours. Reheat gently on the stove or enjoy cold.

Tips for allergens:

Individuals with known allergies or sensitivities to herbal supplements should start with a small amount of Boswellia Tea to ensure no adverse reactions occur. If you are currently taking any medications, consult with a healthcare provider before adding Boswellia Tea to your regimen, as it may interact with certain medications.

68.   Ginger and Turmeric Paste

Beneficial effects:

Ginger and Turmeric Paste combines the powerful anti-inflammatory and antioxidant properties of both ginger and turmeric, making it an effective natural remedy for reducing inflammation, alleviating pain, and boosting the immune system. This paste can be particularly beneficial for individuals suffering from arthritis, digestive issues, and those looking to enhance their overall health and well-being.

Ingredients:

- 1/2 cup of turmeric powder
- 1/4 cup of fresh ginger, grated

- 1 1/2 teaspoons of ground black pepper
- 1/4 cup of coconut oil
- 1/2 cup of water

Instructions:

1. In a small saucepan, combine the turmeric powder, grated ginger, and water. Stir the mixture over low heat until it forms a thick paste.

2. Add the ground black pepper to the mixture. Black pepper increases the bioavailability of curcumin, the active compound in turmeric, enhancing its absorption and effectiveness.

3. Stir in the coconut oil until it is fully integrated into the paste. The fat from the coconut oil also aids in the absorption of turmeric's active compounds.

4. Continue to cook the mixture on low heat for 5-7 minutes, stirring frequently to prevent sticking and ensure even mixing.

5. Once the paste has thickened and the ingredients are well combined, remove from heat and allow it to cool.

Variations:

- For added health benefits, incorporate a teaspoon of cinnamon powder to the paste for its blood sugar-regulating properties.

- If the taste of the paste is too strong, you can add honey to sweeten it naturally when using it in recipes or as a supplement.

Storage tips:

Transfer the cooled paste into a glass jar with a tight-fitting lid and store it in the refrigerator. The paste can be kept for up to 2 weeks. Ensure the jar is clean and dry before storing the paste to prevent mold growth.

Tips for allergens:

Individuals with allergies to ginger or turmeric should proceed with caution and may want to conduct a patch test before applying the paste topically or incorporating it into their diet. For those allergic to coconut oil, olive oil can serve as a suitable substitute, offering similar health benefits and fatty acids essential for the absorption of turmeric.

69.   Holy Basil Tea

Beneficial effects:

Holy Basil Tea, also known as Tulsi Tea, is revered for its powerful adaptogenic and anti-inflammatory properties. It helps in reducing stress, balancing the mind and body, and strengthening the immune system. Consuming Holy Basil Tea can also aid in lowering blood sugar levels, supporting heart health, and providing relief from respiratory disorders.

Ingredients:

- 1 teaspoon of dried Holy Basil leaves
- 1 cup of boiling water
- Honey or lemon (optional, for taste)

Instructions:

1. Place the dried Holy Basil leaves in a tea infuser or directly into a cup.

2. Pour 1 cup of boiling water over the Holy Basil leaves.

3. Cover the cup with a lid or a small plate and allow it to steep for 5 to 10 minutes. The longer

it steeps, the stronger the flavor and therapeutic benefits.

4. Remove the tea infuser or strain the tea to remove the leaves.

5. If desired, add honey or lemon to taste.

6. Enjoy the tea warm, ideally in the morning to start your day or in the evening to unwind.

Variations:

- For a refreshing twist, add a few slices of fresh ginger during the steeping process to enhance its digestive benefits.

- Combine with chamomile flowers for a calming, bedtime tea that promotes relaxation and sleep.

Storage tips:

Store dried Holy Basil leaves in an airtight container in a cool, dark place to maintain their potency and freshness. Prepared Holy Basil Tea is best enjoyed fresh but can be stored in the refrigerator for up to 24 hours. Reheat gently without boiling before consuming.

Tips for allergens:

Individuals with allergies to plants in the Lamiaceae family, such as mint, sage, and oregano, should proceed with caution and may want to consult with a healthcare provider before consuming Holy Basil Tea. If using honey as a sweetener, ensure it's suitable for your dietary needs, especially if you have allergies to bee products.

70. Rosemary Infused Oil

Beneficial effects:

Rosemary Infused Oil harnesses the powerful anti-inflammatory and antioxidant properties of rosemary, making it an excellent natural remedy for improving circulation, relieving pain, and reducing inflammation. Its aromatic compounds also offer stress relief and improved mental clarity.

Ingredients:

- 1 cup of fresh rosemary leaves
- 2 cups of olive oil

Instructions:

1. Wash the rosemary leaves and pat them dry completely to remove any moisture.

2. Place the rosemary leaves in a clean, dry jar.

3. Warm the olive oil in a saucepan over low heat until it is just warm to the touch. Do not allow it to simmer or boil.

4. Pour the warm olive oil over the rosemary leaves, ensuring they are completely submerged.

5. Seal the jar tightly and place it in a sunny spot for 2 to 4 weeks, shaking it gently every few days.

6. After the infusion period, strain the oil through a fine mesh sieve or cheesecloth into a clean, dry bottle. Discard the rosemary leaves.

7. Label the bottle with the contents and date.

Variations:

- For a stronger infusion, add a few cloves of garlic or a sprinkle of dried chili flakes to the jar along with the rosemary leaves before adding the olive oil.

- Combine rosemary with other herbs such as thyme or lavender for additional therapeutic benefits.

Storage tips:

Store the rosemary infused oil in a cool, dark place. When stored properly, it can last up to 6 months. Ensure the bottle is tightly sealed to maintain freshness.

Tips for allergens:

Individuals with allergies to rosemary or olive oil should avoid using this remedy. As an alternative, almond oil or grapeseed oil can be used as the base for those with sensitivities to olive oil.

---

71. Clove and Honey Infusion

Beneficial effects:

Clove and Honey Infusion is a potent remedy known for its anti-inflammatory and antibacterial properties. It can help soothe sore throats, reduce coughing, and boost the immune system. The eugenol in clove oil has been studied for its pain-relieving properties, making this infusion particularly beneficial for those experiencing discomfort from dental issues or minor mouth sores. Honey, on the other hand, acts as a natural cough suppressant and wound healer, further enhancing the soothing effects of the infusion.

Ingredients:

- 1 teaspoon of ground cloves
- 1 cup of boiling water
- 2 tablespoons of raw, organic honey

Instructions:

1. Place the ground cloves in a cup.
2. Pour 1 cup of boiling water over the cloves.
3. Cover the cup and allow it to steep for 10 to 15 minutes. This allows the beneficial compounds in the cloves to infuse into the water.
4. Strain the clove-infused water to remove the ground cloves.
5. Stir in 2 tablespoons of raw, organic honey until it is completely dissolved in the clove-infused water.
6. Consume the infusion while warm for the best soothing effects.

Variations:

- For additional immune support, add a slice of lemon or a teaspoon of lemon juice to the infusion. The vitamin C in lemon can help boost the immune system.
- If you prefer a spicier drink, add a small pinch of ground cinnamon or ginger to the infusion for added warmth and flavor.

Storage tips:

It's best to prepare the Clove and Honey Infusion fresh for each use to maximize its benefits. However, if you need to store it, the infusion (without honey) can be kept in the refrigerator for up to 24 hours. Add honey after reheating gently, just before consumption.

Tips for allergens:

Individuals with allergies to pollen or bee products should proceed with caution when using honey. A high-quality, pure maple syrup can be used as an alternative sweetener, though the texture and flavor of the syrup will differ.

72. Cinnamon and Honey Drink

Beneficial effects:

The Cinnamon and Honey Drink combines the potent anti-inflammatory properties of cinnamon with the antibacterial and soothing benefits of honey, making it an effective natural remedy for reducing inflammation and fighting off colds. This drink can also help in managing blood sugar levels and improving digestion.

Ingredients:

- 1 teaspoon of ground cinnamon
- 1 tablespoon of raw, organic honey
- 1 cup of boiling water

Instructions:

1. Add 1 teaspoon of ground cinnamon to a cup.

2. Pour 1 cup of boiling water over the cinnamon and let it steep for 10 minutes.

3. Strain the mixture to remove any large particles of cinnamon.

4. Stir in 1 tablespoon of raw, organic honey until it dissolves completely.

5. Enjoy the drink warm, preferably on an empty stomach in the morning for digestive benefits or at night for soothing effects before bed.

Variations: -To enhance the anti-inflammatory effects, add a slice of fresh ginger or a pinch of turmeric to the boiling water along with the cinnamon.

- For a refreshing twist, add a few slices of apple to the steeping process, or squeeze in some fresh lemon juice after the drink has been prepared.

Storage tips:

It's best to prepare the Cinnamon and Honey Drink fresh for each use to ensure maximum potency and flavor. However, if you need to prepare it in advance, store it in an airtight container in the refrigerator for up to 24 hours. Reheat gently before consuming.

Tips for allergens:

Individuals with allergies to pollen might react to raw honey. In such cases, substituting honey with maple syrup can provide a similar flavor profile without the allergenic properties. Always ensure that the cinnamon used is pure and not mixed with other spices that could trigger allergies.

73. Black Pepper and Honey Tonic

Beneficial effects:

Black Pepper and Honey Tonic is a potent natural remedy designed to harness the anti-inflammatory and antioxidant properties of black pepper, combined with the soothing and antimicrobial benefits of honey. This tonic is particularly effective in alleviating sore throats, improving digestion, and boosting the immune system. The piperine in black pepper enhances the absorption of curcumin from turmeric and other beneficial compounds, making this tonic a powerful ally in promoting overall health and well-being.

Ingredients:

- 1 teaspoon of freshly ground black pepper
- 2 tablespoons of raw, organic honey
- 1 cup of warm water
- 1/2 teaspoon of turmeric powder (optional, for added anti-inflammatory benefits)

Instructions:

1. Warm 1 cup of water to a comfortable drinking temperature. Avoid boiling to preserve the beneficial enzymes in honey.

2. Add 2 tablespoons of raw, organic honey to the warm water and stir until fully dissolved.

3. Add 1 teaspoon of freshly ground black pepper to the honey-water mixture. Stir well to combine.

4. For added benefits, stir in 1/2 teaspoon of turmeric powder.

5. Consume the tonic immediately, preferably on an empty stomach in the morning to kickstart your digestive system and boost immunity.

Variations:

- To enhance the tonic's soothing effect on sore throats, add a tablespoon of apple cider vinegar.

- For a refreshing twist, squeeze in the juice of half a lemon, which adds vitamin C and further supports immune health.

Storage tips:

This tonic is best prepared fresh to ensure the maximum potency of its ingredients. However, you can prepare a larger batch and store it in the refrigerator for up to 2 days. Ensure it's stored in a clean, airtight glass container.

Tips for allergens:

Individuals with a known allergy to bee products should substitute honey with maple syrup or agave nectar, though the antimicrobial properties may vary. Those with a sensitivity to black pepper can reduce the amount used or consult with a healthcare provider before trying this remedy.

74. Green Tea and Ginger Elixir

Beneficial effects:

The Green Tea and Ginger Elixir harnesses the potent anti-inflammatory and antioxidant properties of green tea combined with the digestive and immune-boosting benefits of ginger. This elixir is ideal for reducing inflammation, supporting immune health, and promoting healthy digestion. Its natural compounds can help soothe sore throats, alleviate nausea, and enhance overall well-being.

Ingredients:

- 1 teaspoon of green tea leaves or 1 green tea bag
- 1-inch piece of fresh ginger, thinly sliced
- 2 cups of boiling water
- Honey or lemon to taste (optional)

Instructions:

1. Place the green tea leaves or tea bag and sliced ginger in a teapot or heatproof pitcher.

2. Pour 2 cups of boiling water over the green tea and ginger.

3. Cover and steep for 3 to 5 minutes, depending on how strong you prefer your tea.

4. Strain the elixir into cups, discarding the tea leaves and ginger slices.

5. If desired, add honey or lemon to taste.

6. Enjoy the elixir warm or let it cool and serve over ice for a refreshing drink.

Variations:

- For an extra immune boost, add a pinch of turmeric to the elixir while it steeps.

- Incorporate a cinnamon stick during the steeping process for added warmth and blood sugar regulation benefits.

Storage tips:

The Green Tea and Ginger Elixir is best enjoyed fresh. However, you can store any leftovers in the refrigerator for up to 24 hours. Reheat gently without boiling or enjoy cold.

Tips for allergens:

Individuals with sensitivities to caffeine should be mindful of the green tea content. For a caffeine-free version, substitute green tea with herbal teas like peppermint or chamomile. If you have allergies to ginger, simply omit it from the recipe.

75. Saffron Milk

Beneficial effects:

Saffron Milk, also known as "Golden Milk," is a traditional remedy known for its potent anti-inflammatory and antioxidant properties. This comforting drink can help reduce inflammation in the body, soothe nerves, and promote a sense of well-being. It's particularly beneficial for improving mood, enhancing sleep quality, and supporting overall immune function.

Ingredients:

- 1 cup of milk (dairy or plant-based)
- 1/4 teaspoon of saffron strands
- 1/2 teaspoon of turmeric powder
- 1/4 teaspoon of ground cinnamon
- 1 teaspoon of honey or maple syrup (optional, for sweetness)
- A pinch of black pepper (to enhance turmeric absorption)

Instructions:

1. Pour the milk into a small saucepan and heat over a low flame until it's warm but not boiling.

2. Add the saffron strands, turmeric powder, ground cinnamon, and a pinch of black pepper to the warm milk.

3. Stir the mixture gently to combine all the ingredients. Allow it to simmer for a few minutes, making sure it doesn't come to a boil.

4. Remove the saucepan from the heat and let the mixture steep for another 2-3 minutes to enhance the flavors.

5. Strain the milk into a cup to remove the saffron strands and any undissolved spices.

6. If desired, sweeten with honey or maple syrup. Stir well.

7. Enjoy the saffron milk warm, preferably before bedtime or when relaxation is needed.

Variations: - For a vegan version, use almond milk, coconut milk, or oat milk as a dairy-free alternative.

- Add a teaspoon of coconut oil or ghee for added richness and to further boost absorption of the turmeric.

- For an extra soothing effect, include a small piece of ginger or a few cardamom pods while heating the milk.

Storage tips:

Saffron Milk is best enjoyed fresh. However, if you need to store it, keep it in the refrigerator in an airtight container for up to 24 hours. Reheat gently before drinking, but do not allow it to boil.

Tips for allergens:

- For those with lactose intolerance or a dairy allergy, ensure to use a plant-based milk that suits your dietary needs.

- If opting for honey as a sweetener, those with allergies to bee products can substitute with maple syrup or agave nectar to avoid any adverse reactions.

Mental Health and Well-being

Mental health and well-being are as crucial to our overall health as physical fitness and proper nutrition. In a world where stress, anxiety, and mood fluctuations have become commonplace, turning to nature's bounty for relief and balance is both empowering and healing. Herbs have been used for centuries not only for their physical healing properties but also for their profound impact on mental health. This section delves into herbal remedies that can support emotional balance, reduce stress, and promote a sense of well-being, offering a natural way to enhance mental health without the side effects often associated with conventional medications.

Objective: To utilize herbal remedies to support mental health and well-being, reducing symptoms of stress, anxiety, and depression naturally.

Preparation:

- Identify specific mental health concerns or areas needing support, such as stress reduction, anxiety relief, or mood improvement.

- Research and select herbs known for their calming, uplifting, or balancing properties.

Materials:

- Herbs such as lavender, chamomile, St. John's Wort, ashwagandha, and lemon balm

- Carrier oils (for making infused oils)

- Alcohol or vinegar (for tinctures)

- Beeswax (if making balms)

- Tea accessories (infusers, teapots, cups)

Tools:

- Jars and bottles for tinctures and oils

- Pots for decoctions and infusions

- Strainer or cheesecloth

- Measuring cups and spoons

Safety measures:

- Verify the safety of each herb, especially if pregnant, nursing, or on medication.

- Start with small doses to monitor body reactions.

Step-by-step instructions:

1. **Lavender Infused Oil for Stress Relief:**

- Gently heat 1 cup of carrier oil and add 1/4 cup of dried lavender flowers.

- Simmer on low heat for 2 hours, ensuring not to boil.

- Strain the oil through cheesecloth into a clean jar. Use by massaging a small amount onto temples or wrists when feeling stressed.

2. **Chamomile Tea for Relaxation**:

- Place 2 teaspoons of dried chamomile flowers into a tea infuser.

- Pour boiling water over the chamomile and steep for 5 minutes.

- Drink in the evening to promote relaxation and support restful sleep.

3. **St. John's Wort Tincture for Mood Support**:

- Fill a jar ⅓ full with dried St. John's Wort and cover with vodka, ensuring herbs are completely submerged.

- Seal the jar and store in a cool, dark place for 6 weeks, shaking daily.

- Strain through cheesecloth and store the tincture in a dark dropper bottle. Use 1-2 ml three times a day to help improve mood.

4. **Ashwagandha Root Decoction for Anxiety**:

- Add 1 teaspoon of dried ashwagandha root to 2 cups of water in a pot.

- Bring to a boil, then simmer for 15 minutes.

- Strain and drink twice daily to help reduce anxiety symptoms.

5. **Lemon Balm and Honey Tea for Cognitive Function**:

- Steep 1 tablespoon of dried lemon balm leaves in 1 cup of boiling water for 10 minutes.

- Strain and add honey to taste. Drink daily to support memory and cognitive function.

Cost estimate: Initial costs may vary depending on the availability of herbs and materials, generally ranging from $20 to $50 for starting supplies.

Time estimate: Preparation times can vary; teas require about 10-15 minutes, while tinctures and infused oils need 4-6 weeks for full potency.

Safety tips:

- Consult with a healthcare provider before starting any herbal regimen, especially for those with pre-existing conditions or those taking medication.

- Always label homemade products with the date made and **Ingredients:** used.

Troubleshooting:

- If a tincture causes irritation, dilute with water or discontinue use.

- If an oil infusion shows signs of mold or spoilage, discard immediately.

Maintenance: Store herbal remedies in a cool, dark place to preserve their potency. Check periodically for any signs of spoilage or degradation.

Difficulty rating: ★☆☆☆☆ to ★★☆☆☆, depending on the complexity of the preparation method.

Variations: Experiment with combining herbs to target multiple aspects of mental health, such as adding peppermint to chamomile tea for both relaxation and improved focus.

By incorporating these herbal remedies into daily routines, individuals can take proactive steps toward enhancing their mental health and well-being. These natural solutions offer a holistic approach to managing stress, anxiety, and mood, providing a gentle yet effective alternative to conventional treatments.

76. Lavender and Chamomile Tea

Beneficial effects:

Lavender and Chamomile Tea is renowned for its calming and soothing properties, making it an excellent natural remedy for managing stress, anxiety, and depression. Lavender has been shown to reduce anxiety and improve sleep quality, while chamomile is known for its mild sedative effects that can help ease the mind and alleviate stress. Together, they create a powerful blend that promotes relaxation and mental well-being.

Ingredients:

- 1 teaspoon of dried lavender flowers
- 1 teaspoon of dried chamomile flowers
- 8 ounces of boiling water
- Honey or lemon (optional, for taste)

Instructions:

1. Place the dried lavender and chamomile flowers in a tea infuser or directly into a cup.

2. Pour 8 ounces of boiling water over the flowers.

3. Cover the cup with a lid or a small plate and let it steep for 5 to 10 minutes. The longer it steeps, the more potent the therapeutic effects.

4. Remove the tea infuser or strain the tea to remove the loose flowers.

5. If desired, add honey or lemon to taste.

6. Enjoy the tea warm, ideally in the evening or whenever relaxation is needed.

Variations:

- For a cooler, refreshing drink, allow the tea to cool to room temperature, then refrigerate for 1-2 hours and serve over ice.
- Add a cinnamon stick or a slice of fresh ginger to the steeping process for added flavor and health benefits.

Storage tips:

Dried lavender and chamomile flowers should be stored in airtight containers in a cool, dark place to maintain their potency and freshness. Prepared tea can be stored in the refrigerator for up to 24 hours. Reheat gently without boiling before consuming.

Tips for allergens:

Individuals with allergies to plants in the Asteraceae family, such as daisies, chrysanthemums, or ragweed, should proceed with caution when consuming chamomile. If you have allergies to bee products, consider using maple syrup or simply enjoy the tea without sweeteners.

77. Valerian Root Tincture

Beneficial effects:

Valerian Root Tincture is renowned for its calming and sedative properties, making it an effective natural remedy for managing stress, anxiety, and depression. It works by increasing the levels of gamma-aminobutyric acid (GABA) in the brain, which helps to regulate nerve cells and calm anxiety. Regular use can improve sleep quality, reduce psychological stress levels, and enhance overall mental well-being.

Ingredients:

- 1/4 cup dried valerian root
- 1 cup vodka or 40% alcohol

Instructions:

1. Place the dried valerian root into a clean, dry jar.

2. Pour the vodka over the valerian root, ensuring that the roots are completely submerged in the alcohol.

3. Seal the jar tightly and label it with the date and contents.

4. Store the jar in a cool, dark place, shaking it daily, for 4 to 6 weeks. This allows the valerian root to infuse the alcohol.

5. After the infusion period, strain the tincture through a cheesecloth or fine mesh strainer into another clean, dry jar, squeezing or pressing the valerian root to extract as much liquid as possible.

6. Label the final product with the date and store it in a cool, dark place.

Variations:

- For a non-alcoholic version, replace vodka with glycerin and water (use a 3:1 ratio of glycerin to water). This variation may have a sweeter taste and a shorter shelf life.

- To enhance the calming effects, consider adding a teaspoon of dried lavender or chamomile flowers to the jar during the infusion process.

Storage tips:

The valerian root tincture should be stored in a cool, dark place, away from direct sunlight. When stored properly, it can last for up to 5 years. Ensure the container is tightly sealed to prevent evaporation and degradation of the active compounds.

Tips for allergens:

Individuals with allergies to valerian root or other plants in the Valerianaceae family should avoid this remedy. Always start with a small dose to ensure no adverse reactions occur, especially if you are trying valerian root for the first time.

78. Passionflower Tea

Beneficial effects:

Passionflower Tea is renowned for its calming and sedative properties, making it an excellent natural remedy for managing stress, anxiety, and depression. Its active compounds, including flavonoids and alkaloids, work synergistically to enhance GABA (gamma-aminobutyric acid) levels in the brain, promoting relaxation and improving sleep quality.

Ingredients:

- 1 tablespoon of dried passionflower
- 1 cup of boiling water
- Honey or lemon (optional, for taste)

Instructions:

1. Place the dried passionflower in a tea infuser or directly into a cup.

2. Pour 1 cup of boiling water over the passionflower.

3. Cover the cup and allow it to steep for 10 to 15 minutes. The longer it steeps, the stronger the tea will be.

4. Remove the tea infuser or strain the tea to remove the loose herbs.

5. If desired, add honey or lemon to taste.

6. Enjoy the tea warm, especially in the evening or whenever relaxation is needed.

Variations:

- For a more potent calming effect, add a teaspoon of dried lavender or chamomile to the infusion.

- To create a soothing bedtime blend, combine passionflower tea with valerian root tea.

Storage tips:

Store dried passionflower in an airtight container in a cool, dark place to maintain its potency. Prepared passionflower tea can be refrigerated in a sealed container for up to 48 hours. Reheat gently without boiling before consuming.

Tips for allergens:

Individuals with allergies to plants in the Passifloraceae family should proceed with caution and may want to consult with a healthcare provider before consuming passionflower tea. If using honey as a sweetener, ensure it's suitable for your dietary needs, especially if you have allergies to bee products.

79. Ashwagandha Smoothie

Beneficial effects:

The Ashwagandha Smoothie is a potent blend designed to manage stress, anxiety, and depression effectively. Ashwagandha, an ancient medicinal herb, is renowned for its adaptogenic properties, helping the body resist stressors of all kinds, whether physical, chemical, or biological. This smoothie combines the stress-reducing power of ashwagandha with the nutritional benefits of other ingredients to promote overall well-being and mental health.

Portions

Serves 2

Preparation time

5 minutes

Ingredients:

- 2 teaspoons of ashwagandha powder
- 1 ripe banana
- 1/2 cup of blueberries (fresh or frozen)
- 1 cup of spinach leaves
- 1 tablespoon of flaxseeds
- 1 cup of almond milk (unsweetened)
- 1 tablespoon of honey (optional, for sweetness)

Instructions:

1. Place the ashwagandha powder, ripe banana, blueberries, spinach leaves, and flaxseeds into a blender.

2. Add the almond milk to the blender.

3. Blend on high until the mixture is smooth and creamy.

4. Taste the smoothie and, if desired, add honey for additional sweetness. Blend again for a few seconds to incorporate the honey.

5. Pour the smoothie into two glasses and serve immediately.

Variations:

- For an extra protein boost, add a scoop of your favorite plant-based protein powder before blending.

- Substitute almond milk with coconut water or any other nut milk of your choice for a different flavor profile.

- Add a pinch of cinnamon or nutmeg for added warmth and spice.

Storage tips:

This smoothie is best enjoyed fresh. However, if you need to store it, keep it in an airtight container in the refrigerator for up to 24 hours. Shake well before consuming if ingredients have settled.

Tips for allergens:

If you have a nut allergy, substitute almond milk with oat milk or another non-nut-based milk alternative. Always ensure that the ashwagandha powder used is pure and free from any additives that could cause allergic reactions.

80. Lemon Balm and Honey Infusion

Beneficial effects:

Lemon Balm and Honey Infusion is a calming herbal remedy known for its ability to reduce stress, anxiety, and symptoms of depression. Lemon balm, with its mild sedative properties, promotes relaxation and improves mood, while honey adds a soothing and comforting effect. This infusion is particularly beneficial for those looking to ease nervous tension and achieve a state of calmness and well-being.

Ingredients

- 2 tablespoons of dried lemon balm leaves
- 1 tablespoon of raw, organic honey
- 1 cup of boiling water

Instructions:

1. Place the dried lemon balm leaves in a tea infuser or directly into a cup.

2. Pour 1 cup of boiling water over the lemon balm leaves.

3. Cover the cup and allow it to steep for 10 minutes.

4. Remove the tea infuser or strain the tea to remove the leaves.

5. Stir in 1 tablespoon of raw, organic honey until it dissolves completely.

6. Enjoy the infusion warm, ideally in the evening to unwind before bed or any time during the day when stress relief is needed.

Variations:

- For an added boost of flavor and health benefits, include a slice of fresh ginger or a few leaves of fresh mint to the infusion while it steeps.

- If you prefer a cooler beverage, allow the tea to cool to room temperature, then refrigerate for 1-2 hours and serve over ice.

Storage tips:

This infusion is best enjoyed fresh. However, if you need to store it, keep it in the refrigerator in a tightly sealed container for up to 24 hours. Reheat gently without boiling before consuming.

Tips for allergens:

Individuals with allergies to plants in the mint family should proceed with caution when using lemon balm. If you have allergies to bee products, you can omit the honey or substitute it with maple syrup for a similar sweetening effect without the allergenic properties.

81. Rhodiola Rosea Capsules

Beneficial effects:

Rhodiola Rosea Capsules offer a natural way to manage stress, anxiety, and depression. Known for its adaptogenic properties, Rhodiola Rosea helps the body adapt to and resist physical, chemical, and environmental stress. By improving mood and alleviating stress symptoms, these capsules can enhance overall well-being and mental health.

Ingredients

- 400 mg of Rhodiola Rosea extract (standardized to contain 3% rosavins and 1% salidroside)

- Vegetable capsule shells

Instructions:

1. Measure 400 mg of Rhodiola Rosea extract using a digital scale for accuracy.

2. Carefully open a vegetable capsule shell and fill the larger end with the measured Rhodiola Rosea extract.

3. Once filled, cap the capsule with the smaller end, pressing firmly to ensure it's securely closed.

4. Repeat the process for the desired number of capsules.

Dosage

Take one capsule in the morning on an empty stomach, 30 minutes before breakfast. If well tolerated, an additional capsule may be taken early in the afternoon or as directed by a healthcare professional.

Variations:

- For enhanced stress-relief effects, consider combining Rhodiola Rosea capsules with other adaptogenic herbs such as Ashwagandha or Holy Basil in your regimen.

- Individuals sensitive to Rhodiola Rosea may start with a half dose (200 mg) to assess tolerance before gradually increasing to the full dose.

Storage tips:

Store the prepared Rhodiola Rosea capsules in a cool, dry place, away from direct sunlight and moisture. Ensure the container is airtight to maintain the potency of the extract.

Tips for allergens:

- Individuals with allergies to plants in the Crassulaceae family should proceed with caution and may want to consult with a healthcare provider before taking Rhodiola Rosea capsules.

- Ensure the vegetable capsule shells are free from allergens that may affect you, such as soy or gluten, by checking the product label if you're purchasing them separately.

82. Holy Basil and Mint Tea

Beneficial effects:

Holy Basil and Mint Tea is a soothing and refreshing beverage that harnesses the adaptogenic properties of Holy Basil (Tulsi) along with the digestive benefits of mint. This tea is particularly beneficial for managing stress, anxiety, and depression, promoting a sense of calm and well-being. Holy Basil is known for its ability to lower cortisol levels, thus reducing stress, while mint can help soothe the stomach and improve digestion, contributing to overall relaxation and balance.

Ingredients:

- 1 tablespoon of dried Holy Basil leaves
- 1 tablespoon of dried mint leaves
- 2 cups of boiling water
- Honey or lemon to taste (optional)

Instructions:

1. Place the dried Holy Basil leaves and dried mint leaves in a tea infuser or directly into a teapot.
2. Pour 2 cups of boiling water over the leaves.
3. Cover and allow the tea to steep for 5 to 10 minutes, depending on the desired strength.
4. Remove the tea infuser or strain the tea to remove the leaves.
5. If desired, add honey or lemon to taste.
6. Serve the tea warm for immediate comfort or allow it to cool and enjoy it as a refreshing cold beverage.

Variations:

- For a caffeine boost that can also aid in concentration, add a green tea bag to the infusion process.

- Incorporate a slice of fresh ginger for additional digestive and anti-inflammatory benefits.

Storage tips:

If you have leftover tea, it can be stored in a sealed container in the refrigerator for up to 2 days. Enjoy it cold, or gently reheat it without bringing it to a boil.

Tips for allergens:

Individuals with specific plant allergies should ensure they are not allergic to Holy Basil or mint before consuming this tea. For those avoiding honey due to allergies or vegan preferences, stevia or agave syrup can serve as alternative sweeteners.

83. Skullcap Tincture

Beneficial effects:

Skullcap Tincture is renowned for its calming and neuroprotective properties, making it an effective natural remedy for managing stress, anxiety, and depression. It acts on the nervous system to promote relaxation, reduce tension, and improve mood. The bioactive compounds in skullcap, such as baicalin, have been shown to enhance neurotransmitter levels in the brain, contributing to its soothing effects.

Ingredients:

- 1/4 cup dried skullcap herb
- 1 cup high-proof alcohol (vodka or grain alcohol is suitable)

Instructions:

1. Place the dried skullcap herb into a clean, dry glass jar.
2. Pour the high-proof alcohol over the herbs, ensuring they are completely submerged.
3. Seal the jar tightly and label it with the date and contents.
4. Store the jar in a cool, dark place, shaking it daily, for 4 to 6 weeks. This allows the alcohol to extract the active compounds from the skullcap.
5. After the infusion period, strain the tincture through a cheesecloth or fine mesh strainer into another clean, dry jar, pressing the herbs to extract as much liquid as possible.
6. Label the final product with the date and store it in a cool, dark place.

Variations:

- For those sensitive to alcohol, a glycerin-based tincture can be made by substituting alcohol with a mixture of glycerin and water (use a 3:1 ratio of glycerin to water).
- Combine skullcap with other calming herbs such as chamomile or lavender in the tincture to enhance its stress-relieving effects.

Storage tips:

The skullcap tincture should be stored in a cool, dark place, away from direct sunlight. When stored properly, it can last for several years. Ensure the container is tightly sealed to prevent evaporation and maintain potency.

Tips for allergens:

Individuals with known allergies or sensitivities to skullcap or other herbs should start with a small dose to assess tolerance. Always consult with a healthcare provider before adding new herbal remedies to your regimen, especially if you are pregnant, nursing, or taking medication.

84. Kava Kava Tea

Beneficial effects:

Kava Kava Tea is renowned for its calming and therapeutic effects, making it an excellent natural remedy for managing stress, anxiety, and depression. The active **Ingredients:** in Kava, known as kavalactones, have been shown to promote relaxation, improve mood, and enhance cognitive function without impairing mental clarity.

Ingredients:

- 1 teaspoon of ground Kava root
- 1 cup of boiling water
- Honey or lemon (optional, for taste)

Instructions:

1. Place the ground Kava root in a tea infuser or directly into a cup.

2. Pour 1 cup of boiling water over the Kava root.

3. Allow the tea to steep for 5 to 10 minutes. The longer it steeps, the stronger the effects will be.

4. Remove the tea infuser or strain the tea to remove the ground root.

5. If desired, add honey or lemon to taste.

6. Enjoy the Kava Kava Tea in the evening or when relaxation is needed. Due to its potent effects, start with one cup to assess your tolerance.

Variations:

- For a creamier texture and added flavor, blend the strained tea with coconut milk and a pinch of cinnamon or nutmeg.

- Combine Kava Kava Tea with chamomile or lavender tea for additional relaxing and sleep-promoting benefits.

Storage tips:

Store ground Kava root in an airtight container in a cool, dark place to maintain its potency. It is best to prepare Kava Kava Tea fresh for each use to ensure maximum effectiveness and flavor.

Tips for allergens:

Individuals with allergies to Kava should avoid this remedy. As Kava can interact with certain medications and conditions, consult with a healthcare provider before incorporating it into your routine, especially if you are pregnant, nursing, or taking medications for anxiety or depression.

85. St. John's Wort Tea

Beneficial effects:

St. John's Wort Tea is renowned for its natural mood-lifting properties, making it a valuable herbal remedy for managing stress, anxiety, and mild to moderate depression. The active compounds in St. John's Wort, such as hypericin and hyperforin, are thought to influence neurotransmitters in the brain that are involved in mood regulation. This herbal tea can help promote a sense of calm and well-being, making it an excellent choice for those looking to naturally support their mental health.

Ingredients:

- 1 to 2 teaspoons of dried St. John's Wort

- 8 ounces of boiling water

- Honey or lemon (optional, for taste)

Instructions:

1. Place the dried St. John's Wort in a tea infuser or directly into a cup.

2. Pour 8 ounces of boiling water over the St. John's Wort.

3. Cover the cup with a lid or a small plate and let it steep for 5 to 10 minutes. The longer it steeps, the more potent the tea will be.

4. Remove the tea infuser or strain the tea to remove the loose herbs.

5. If desired, add honey or lemon to taste.

6. Enjoy the tea warm, ideally in the morning to start your day or in the evening to unwind.

Variations:

- For added relaxation benefits, combine St. John's Wort with chamomile or lavender in your tea blend.

- If you prefer a cooler beverage, allow the tea to cool to room temperature, then refrigerate for 1-2 hours and serve over ice.

Storage tips:

Store dried St. John's Wort in a cool, dry place away from direct sunlight to preserve its potency and flavor. Prepared St. John's Wort tea can be refrigerated in a sealed container for up to 24 hours. Reheat gently without boiling before consuming.

Tips for allergens:

Individuals with known sensitivities to plants in the Hypericaceae family should start with a small amount of St. John's Wort tea to ensure no adverse reactions occur. If using honey as a sweetener, ensure it's suitable for your dietary needs, especially if you have allergies to bee products.

Calming Teas and Tinctures

Creating calming teas and tinctures can be a soothing and effective way to manage stress, anxiety, and improve overall well-being. These herbal remedies harness the natural properties of plants to help calm the mind, soothe the nerves, and promote relaxation. With a focus on simplicity and accessibility, this section guides you through the process of making your own calming teas and tinctures at home, using ingredients that are both easy to find and gentle on the body.

Objective: To prepare natural, calming herbal teas and tinctures that support relaxation and stress relief.

Preparation:

- Choose herbs known for their calming effects, such as chamomile, lavender, lemon balm, passionflower, and valerian root.

- Decide whether you want to create a tea for immediate use or a tincture for longer-term storage.

Materials:

- Dried herbs of choice

- Water (for teas)

- High-proof alcohol (for tinctures) or apple cider vinegar/glycerin (for non-alcoholic tinctures)

- Glass jars with tight-fitting lids (for tinctures)

- Teapot or saucepan (for teas)

Tools:

- Strainer or cheesecloth

- Measuring cups and spoons

- Funnel (for tinctures)

- Labels and marker

Safety measures:

- Ensure all herbs are correctly identified and sourced from reputable suppliers.

- Start with small doses to test for personal sensitivities.

Step-by-step Instructions:

1. **Chamomile Tea**:

- Boil 1 cup of water.

- Add 2 teaspoons of dried chamomile flowers to the boiling water.

- Steep for 5-10 minutes, then strain.

- Enjoy warm, adding honey if desired for sweetness.

2. **Lavender Tincture**:

- Fill a glass jar ⅓ full with dried lavender flowers.

- Cover the flowers with high-proof alcohol, ensuring they are completely submerged.

- Seal the jar and label it with the date and contents.

- Store in a cool, dark place for 4-6 weeks, shaking the jar daily.

- After 4-6 weeks, strain the liquid through a cheesecloth into a clean bottle. Label the bottle.

3. **Lemon Balm Tea**:

- Boil 1 cup of water.

- Add 1 tablespoon of dried lemon balm leaves to the boiling water.

- Steep for 5-10 minutes, then strain.

- Drink as needed to promote calm and relaxation.

4. **Passionflower Tincture**:

- Repeat the steps for the lavender tincture, substituting dried passionflower for lavender.

Cost estimate: Costs vary depending on the herbs and materials used but generally range from $10 to $30 for starting supplies.

Time estimate:

- Teas are ready in about 10-15 minutes.

- Tinctures require 4-6 weeks for full extraction.

Safety tips:

- Consult with a healthcare professional before using herbal remedies, especially if pregnant, nursing, or taking other medications.

- Label all homemade products clearly with ingredients and dates.

Troubleshooting:

- If a tea is too strong, dilute with more water.

- If a tincture is too weak, allow it to steep for a longer period or add more herbs initially.

Maintenance:

- Store teas in a cool, dry place and use within a year.

- Tinctures, when stored properly in a cool, dark place, can last for several years.

Difficulty rating: ★☆☆☆☆. Making teas and tinctures is straightforward and suitable for beginners.

Variations:

- Experiment with combining herbs to create custom blends tailored to your taste and relaxation needs.

- For non-alcoholic tinctures, use glycerin or apple cider vinegar as a solvent, following the same steps as for alcohol-based tinctures.

By incorporating these calming teas and tinctures into your routine, you can enjoy a natural and gentle way to unwind and de-stress. Whether you prefer the immediate soothing effect of a warm cup of herbal tea or the convenience of a tincture for on-the-go support, these remedies offer a holistic approach to relaxation and mental well-being.

86. *Echinacea Tincture*

Beneficial effects:

Echinacea Tincture is a powerful immune system booster, known for its ability to enhance the body's natural defense mechanisms against common colds, flu, and other respiratory infections. Its active compounds, including alkamides, polysaccharides, and glycoproteins, have been shown to stimulate immune function, reduce inflammation, and accelerate recovery time.

Ingredients:

- 1/4 cup dried Echinacea purpurea root
- 1/2 cup 100-proof vodka

Instructions:

1. Place the dried Echinacea root into a clean, dry jar.

2. Pour the vodka over the Echinacea, ensuring the roots are completely submerged. Add more vodka if necessary.

3. Seal the jar tightly and label it with the date and contents.

4. Store the jar in a cool, dark place, shaking it daily, for 4 to 6 weeks. This allows the Echinacea to infuse the vodka.

5. After the infusion period, strain the tincture through a cheesecloth or fine mesh strainer into another clean, dry jar, pressing the Echinacea to extract as much liquid as possible.

6. Transfer the strained tincture into a dark glass dropper bottle for easy use.

Variations:

- For a non-alcoholic version, glycerin can be substituted for vodka, creating a glycerite. Use a 3:1 ratio of glycerin to water for the infusion.
- Combine Echinacea with other immune-boosting herbs such as elderberry or astragalus for a comprehensive immune support tincture.

Storage tips:

Store the Echinacea Tincture in a cool, dark place, such as a cabinet. When stored properly, the tincture can last for up to 5 years. Ensure the dropper bottle is tightly sealed to maintain potency.

Tips for allergens:

Individuals with allergies to plants in the daisy family should proceed with caution when using Echinacea. Always consult with a healthcare provider before beginning any new herbal supplement, especially if you have a known allergy or are taking other medications.

87. Astragalus Root Tea

Beneficial effects:

Astragalus Root Tea is celebrated for its immune-boosting properties, making it an essential remedy for enhancing the body's defense mechanisms. This herbal tea stimulates the immune system, promoting overall health and protecting against common illnesses. Its antioxidant properties also help to combat oxidative stress, supporting the body's natural resilience.

Ingredients:

- 1 tablespoon of dried astragalus root
- 2 cups of water

Instructions:

1. Add 2 cups of water and 1 tablespoon of dried astragalus root to a small saucepan.

2. Bring the mixture to a boil, then reduce the heat and simmer for about 20 minutes. This slow cooking process allows the water to become infused with the astragalus root's beneficial properties.

3. After simmering, strain the tea into a cup or mug, removing the astragalus root pieces.

4. Enjoy the tea warm, ideally once in the morning and once in the evening to support your immune system.

Variations:

- To enhance the flavor and add additional health benefits, consider adding a slice of ginger or a stick of cinnamon to the tea while it simmers.

- For a sweeter taste, stir in a teaspoon of honey after removing the tea from heat.

Storage tips:

Prepare astragalus root tea fresh for each use to ensure maximum potency and benefits. However, if you need to store the tea, keep it in a sealed container in the refrigerator for up to 24 hours. Reheat gently on the stove before consuming.

Tips for allergens:

Individuals with allergies to legumes should consult with a healthcare provider before consuming astragalus root tea, as astragalus is a member of the legume family. If adding honey, those with allergies to bee products can substitute it with maple syrup or simply enjoy the tea without sweeteners.

88. Reishi Mushroom Soup

Beneficial effects:

Reishi Mushroom Soup is a nourishing and immune-boosting remedy, perfect for enhancing the body's defense mechanisms. Reishi mushrooms are celebrated for their ability to support immune health, reduce stress, and improve sleep quality. This soup combines the medicinal properties of Reishi with other healthful ingredients to create a delicious and therapeutic dish.

Portions

Serves 4

Preparation time

15 minutes

Cooking time

1 hour

Ingredients:

- 4 cups of vegetable broth
- 1 cup of Reishi mushrooms, sliced
- 1 cup of shiitake mushrooms, sliced
- 1 medium onion, chopped
- 2 cloves of garlic, minced
- 1 carrot, chopped
- 1 stalk of celery, chopped
- 1 teaspoon of grated ginger
- 2 tablespoons of olive oil
- Salt and pepper to taste
- Fresh parsley for garnish (optional)

Instructions:

1. In a large pot, heat the olive oil over medium heat.

2. Add the chopped onion, garlic, and ginger to the pot and sauté until the onion becomes translucent, about 5 minutes.

3. Add the Reishi and shiitake mushrooms to the pot and cook for another 5 minutes, stirring occasionally.

4. Add the chopped carrot and celery to the pot and sauté for a few more minutes.

5. Pour the vegetable broth into the pot and bring the mixture to a boil.

6. Reduce the heat to low and let the soup simmer for about 45 minutes to an hour, allowing the flavors to meld and the Reishi mushrooms to release their medicinal properties.

7. Season the soup with salt and pepper to taste.

8. Serve the soup hot, garnished with fresh parsley if desired.

Variations:

- For added protein, include a cup of cooked quinoa or chickpeas in the soup.
- To enhance the immune-boosting properties, stir in a teaspoon of turmeric powder along with the vegetable broth.
- For a creamy texture, blend half of the soup and then combine it with the remaining chunky soup before serving.

Storage tips:

Store any leftover soup in an airtight container in the refrigerator for up to 3 days. Reheat on the stove or in the microwave before serving. The soup can also be frozen for up to 3 months. Thaw in the refrigerator overnight and reheat thoroughly.

Tips for allergens:

For those with allergies to mushrooms, it's essential to consult with a healthcare provider before trying Reishi mushroom soup. The recipe can be adapted by omitting the Reishi and shiitake mushrooms and focusing on the broth and vegetables for a simple yet nutritious alternative.

89. Elderberry and Echinacea Syrup

Beneficial effects:

Elderberry and Echinacea Syrup combines the immune-boosting power of elderberries with the anti-inflammatory benefits of echinacea, creating a potent remedy for preventing and fighting off colds and flu. Elderberries are rich in antioxidants and vitamins that can boost your immune system, while echinacea is known for its ability to enhance the body's natural defense mechanism. Together, they form a powerful duo that can shorten the duration of colds, alleviate symptoms, and protect against respiratory infections.

Portions

Makes approximately 16 ounces

Preparation time

10 minutes

Cooking time

30 minutes

Ingredients:

- 3/4 cup dried elderberries
- 1/2 cup echinacea purpurea root
- 4 cups water
- 1 cup raw honey
- 2 tablespoons fresh ginger, grated
- 1 cinnamon stick
- 1 teaspoon whole cloves

Instructions:

1. Combine the dried elderberries, echinacea root, fresh ginger, cinnamon stick, and whole cloves with water in a medium saucepan.

2. Bring the mixture to a boil, then reduce the heat and simmer for about 30 minutes, or until the liquid has reduced by half.

3. Remove from heat and let the mixture cool until it is safe to handle.

4. Mash the berries and echinacea root using a spoon or potato masher to release any additional juice.

5. Strain the mixture through a fine mesh strainer or cheesecloth into a large bowl, pressing on the solids to extract as much liquid as possible. Discard the solids.

6. Once the liquid has cooled to lukewarm, add the raw honey and stir until it is well incorporated.

7. Pour the syrup into sterilized glass bottles or jars.

Variations:

- For additional respiratory support, add a teaspoon of dried thyme or peppermint leaves during the simmering process.

- If you prefer a vegan version, substitute honey with maple syrup or agave nectar, adjusting the sweetness to your taste.

Storage tips:

Store the Elderberry and Echinacea Syrup in the refrigerator for up to 3 months. For longer shelf life, you can freeze the syrup in an ice cube tray and then transfer the cubes to a freezer bag for easy dosage.

Tips for allergens:

For those with allergies to honey, maple syrup or agave nectar are suitable alternatives that do not compromise the syrup's effectiveness.

If you have a known allergy to echinacea, elderberry, or any of the other ingredients, please consult with a healthcare provider before using this remedy.

90. Garlic and Ginger Immune Boosting Soup

Beneficial effects:

Garlic and Ginger Immune Boosting Soup combines the powerful immune-supporting properties of garlic and ginger with the nourishing benefits of vegetables and chicken broth. Garlic has natural antibacterial and antiviral properties, while ginger is known for its anti-inflammatory effects. Together, they create a potent remedy to help ward off colds, flu, and other infections, promoting overall immune system health.

Portions

Serves 4

Preparation time

15 minutes

Cooking time

1 hour

Ingredients:

- 4 cups of chicken broth
- 2 cups of water
- 1 chicken breast (optional, can be omitted for a vegetarian version)
- 1 cup of chopped carrots
- 1 cup of chopped celery
- 4 cloves of garlic, minced
- 1 inch of fresh ginger, grated
- 1 onion, chopped
- 1 teaspoon of turmeric powder
- Salt and pepper to taste
- 2 tablespoons of olive oil
- Fresh parsley for garnish

Instructions:

1. Heat the olive oil in a large pot over medium heat.

2. Add the chopped onion, carrots, and celery. Sauté until the vegetables are slightly softened, about 5 minutes.

3. Add the minced garlic and grated ginger, and cook for another 2 minutes until fragrant.

4. Pour in the chicken broth and water, then add the chicken breast to the pot (if using).

5. Stir in the turmeric powder, and season with salt and pepper.

6. Bring the soup to a boil, then reduce the heat to low and simmer, covered, for about 45 minutes to 1 hour, or until the chicken is cooked through and the vegetables are tender.

7. If using chicken, remove it from the pot, shred it with two forks, and return it to the soup.

8. Adjust the seasoning if necessary.

9. Serve the soup hot, garnished with fresh parsley.

Variations:

- For a vegetarian version, omit the chicken and use vegetable broth instead of chicken broth.

- Add other immune-boosting ingredients like spinach, kale, or mushrooms for added nutrients.

- For a spicy kick, add a pinch of cayenne pepper or a few slices of fresh jalapeño.

Storage tips:

Store any leftovers in an airtight container in the refrigerator for up to 3 days. Reheat on the stove or in the microwave until hot. This soup can also be frozen for up to 3 months. Thaw in the refrigerator overnight before reheating.

Tips for allergens:

For those with allergies to chicken, ensure to use the vegetarian version of this recipe. If you're sensitive to garlic or ginger, adjust the amounts according to your tolerance or consult with a healthcare provider before consuming.

91. *Elderberry and Echinacea Syrup*

Beneficial effects:

Elderberry and Echinacea Syrup is a powerful combination designed to boost the immune system. Elderberry is packed with antioxidants and vitamins that can help fight inflammation and lessen stress on the body, while echinacea is known for its ability to enhance the body's immune response. Together, they create a potent natural remedy for preventing and fighting off colds, flu, and other respiratory infections.

Portions

Makes approximately 2 cups

Preparation time

15 minutes

Cooking time

45 minutes to 1 hour

Ingredients:

- 3/4 cup dried elderberries
- 1/2 cup dried echinacea purpurea leaves and flowers
- 4 cups water
- 1 cup raw honey
- 2 tablespoons fresh grated ginger
- 1 cinnamon stick
- 1 teaspoon whole cloves

Instructions:

1. Combine elderberries, echinacea, ginger, cinnamon stick, and cloves with water in a medium saucepan.

2. Bring the mixture to a boil, then reduce heat and simmer, covered, until the liquid is reduced by half, about 45 minutes to 1 hour.

3. Remove from heat and let cool until it is safe to handle.

4. Mash the berries and echinacea slightly to release their juices.

5. Strain the mixture through a fine mesh strainer or cheesecloth into a large bowl, pressing to extract as much liquid as possible. Discard the solids.

6. Allow the liquid to cool to lukewarm, then stir in the raw honey until well combined.

7. Transfer the syrup to sterilized glass bottles or jars.

Variations:

- For a vegan version, substitute honey with maple syrup or agave nectar.

- Add a few drops of lemon juice for additional vitamin C and a tangy flavor.

- Incorporate a sprig of thyme or rosemary during the simmering process for added respiratory benefits.

Storage tips:

Store the syrup in the refrigerator for up to 3 months. For extended storage, freeze in an airtight container or ice cube trays for easy dosing, and use within 6 months.

Tips for allergens:

If you are allergic to any of the ingredients, consult with a healthcare provider before using. Honey should not be given to children under 1 year of age due to the risk of botulism.

92. Garlic and Ginger Immune Boosting Soup

Beneficial effects:

Garlic and Ginger Immune Boosting Soup is designed to strengthen the immune system, thanks to the powerful combination of garlic and ginger, both of which are renowned for their antibacterial, antiviral, and anti-inflammatory properties. This hearty soup also incorporates a variety of vegetables and chicken broth to nourish the body and provide essential nutrients, making it an ideal remedy for cold and flu season.

Portions

Serves 4

Preparation time

15 minutes

Cooking time

1 hour

Ingredients:

- 4 cups of chicken broth
- 2 cups of water
- 1 chicken breast (optional, can be omitted for a vegetarian version)
- 1 cup of chopped carrots
- 1 cup of chopped celery
- 4 cloves of garlic, minced
- 1 inch of fresh ginger, grated
- 1 onion, chopped
- 1 teaspoon of turmeric powder
- Salt and pepper to taste
- 2 tablespoons of olive oil
- Fresh parsley for garnish

Instructions:

1. In a large pot, heat the olive oil over medium heat.

2. Add the chopped onion, carrots, and celery. Sauté until the vegetables are slightly softened, about 5 minutes.

3. Add the minced garlic and grated ginger, and cook for another 2 minutes until fragrant.

4. Pour in the chicken broth and water, then add the chicken breast to the pot (if using).

5. Stir in the turmeric powder, and season with salt and pepper.

6. Bring the soup to a boil, then reduce the heat to low and simmer, covered, for about 45 minutes to 1 hour, or until the chicken is cooked through and the vegetables are tender.

7. If using chicken, remove it from the pot, shred it with two forks, and return it to the soup.

8. Adjust the seasoning if necessary.

9. Serve the soup hot, garnished with fresh parsley.

Variations:

- For a vegan version, omit the chicken and use vegetable broth instead of chicken broth.
- Add other immune-boosting ingredients like spinach, kale, or mushrooms for added nutrients.
- For a spicy kick, add a pinch of cayenne pepper or a few slices of fresh jalapeño.

Storage tips: Store any leftovers in an airtight container in the refrigerator for up to

3 days. Reheat on the stove or in the microwave until hot. This soup can also be frozen for up to 3 months. Thaw in the refrigerator overnight before reheating.

Tips for allergens

For those with allergies to chicken, ensure to use the vegetarian version of this recipe. If you're sensitive to garlic or ginger, adjust the amounts according to your tolerance or consult with a healthcare provider before consuming.

93. Astragalus Root Tea

Beneficial effects:

Astragalus Root Tea is a traditional remedy known for its immune-boosting properties. It helps to strengthen the body's defense mechanisms against common colds, flu, and other infections. Astragalus is also believed to increase energy levels and support overall vitality, making it an excellent choice for those looking to naturally enhance their immune system and promote a sense of well-being.

Ingredients:

- 1 tablespoon of dried astragalus root
- 2 cups of water

Instructions:

1. Add 2 cups of water and 1 tablespoon of dried astragalus root to a small saucepan.

2. Bring the mixture to a boil, then reduce the heat and simmer for about 20 minutes. This slow cooking process allows the water to become infused with the astragalus root's beneficial properties.

3. After simmering, strain the tea into a cup or mug, removing the astragalus root pieces.

4. Enjoy the tea warm, ideally once in the morning and once in the evening to support your immune system.

Variations:

- To enhance the flavor and add additional health benefits, consider adding a slice of ginger or a stick of cinnamon to the tea while it simmers.

- For a sweeter taste, stir in a teaspoon of honey after removing the tea from heat.

Storage tips:

Prepare astragalus root tea fresh for each use to ensure maximum potency and benefits. However, if you need to store the tea, keep it in a sealed container in the refrigerator for up to 24 hours. Reheat gently on the stove before consuming.

Tips for allergens:

Individuals with allergies to legumes should consult with a healthcare provider before consuming astragalus root tea, as astragalus is a member of the legume family. If adding honey, those with allergies to bee products can substitute it with maple syrup or simply enjoy the tea without sweeteners.

94. Reishi Mushroom Soup

Beneficial effects:

Reishi Mushroom Soup is a powerful immune-boosting remedy, incorporating the medicinal properties of Reishi mushrooms which are known for enhancing the immune system, reducing stress, and improving sleep quality. This soup not only nourishes the body but also provides a natural way to support overall health and well-being.

Portions

Serves 4

Preparation time

15 minutes

Cooking time

1 hour

Ingredients:

- 4 cups of vegetable broth
- 1 cup of Reishi mushrooms, sliced
- 1 cup of shiitake mushrooms, sliced
- 1 medium onion, chopped
- 2 cloves of garlic, minced
- 1 carrot, chopped
- 1 stalk of celery, chopped
- 1 teaspoon of grated ginger
- 2 tablespoons of olive oil
- Salt and pepper to taste
- Fresh parsley for garnish (optional)

Instructions:

1. In a large pot, heat the olive oil over medium heat.

2. Add the chopped onion, garlic, and ginger to the pot and sauté until the onion becomes translucent, about 5 minutes.

3. Add the Reishi and shiitake mushrooms to the pot and cook for another 5 minutes, stirring occasionally.

4. Add the chopped carrot and celery to the pot and sauté for a few more minutes.

5. Pour the vegetable broth into the pot and bring the mixture to a boil.

6. Reduce the heat to low and let the soup simmer for about 45 minutes to an hour, allowing the flavors to meld and the Reishi mushrooms to release their medicinal properties.

7. Season the soup with salt and pepper to taste.

8. Serve the soup hot, garnished with fresh parsley if desired.

Variations:

- For added protein, include a cup of cooked quinoa or chickpeas in the soup.
- To enhance the immune-boosting properties, stir in a teaspoon of turmeric powder along with the vegetable broth.
- For a creamy texture, blend half of the soup and then combine it with the remaining chunky soup before serving.

Storage tips:

Store any leftover soup in an airtight container in the refrigerator for up to 3 days. Reheat on the stove or in the microwave before serving. The soup can also be frozen for up to 3 months. Thaw in the refrigerator overnight and reheat thoroughly.

Tips for allergens: For those with allergies to mushrooms, it's essential to consult with a healthcare provider before trying Reishi mushroom soup. The recipe can be adapted by omitting the Reishi and shiitake mushrooms and focusing on the broth and vegetables for a simple yet nutritious alternative.

95. Echinacea Tincture

Beneficial effects:

Echinacea Tincture is a natural remedy known for its ability to boost the immune system, helping to fend off colds, flu, and other respiratory infections. Its active compounds, including alkamides, polysaccharides, and glycoproteins, support immune function and have anti-inflammatory properties. Regular use can shorten the duration of illnesses and may reduce the severity of symptoms.

Ingredients:

- 1/4 cup dried Echinacea purpurea root
- 1/2 cup 100-proof alcohol (vodka or grain alcohol)

Instructions:

1. Place the dried Echinacea root into a clean, dry jar.

2. Pour the alcohol over the Echinacea, ensuring the roots are completely submerged. Add more alcohol if necessary.

3. Seal the jar tightly and label it with the date and contents.

4. Store the jar in a cool, dark place, shaking it daily, for 4 to 6 weeks. This allows the Echinacea to infuse the alcohol.

5. After the infusion period, strain the tincture through a cheesecloth or fine mesh strainer into another clean, dry jar, pressing the Echinacea to extract as much liquid as possible.

6. Transfer the strained tincture into a dark glass dropper bottle for easy use.

Variations:

- For those sensitive to alcohol, replace vodka with a glycerin and water mixture (3:1 ratio of glycerin to water) to create a non-alcoholic tincture.

- Combine Echinacea with other immune-supporting herbs such as elderberry or astragalus in the tincture for a comprehensive immune-boosting remedy.

Storage tips:

Store the Echinacea Tincture in a cool, dark place. When stored properly, the tincture can last for up to 5 years. Ensure the dropper bottle is tightly sealed to maintain potency.

Tips for allergens:

Individuals with allergies to plants in the daisy family should proceed with caution and may want to consult with a healthcare provider before using Echinacea. Always start with a small dose to ensure no adverse reactions occur.

96. *Elderberry and Nettle Tonic*

Beneficial effects:

Elderberry and Nettle Tonic is a powerful blend designed to strengthen the immune system and alleviate allergy symptoms. Elderberries are rich in vitamins and antioxidants that support immune health, while nettle is known for its natural antihistamine properties, helping to ease seasonal allergy symptoms. This tonic is ideal for those looking to naturally boost their immune system and reduce the impact of allergies.

Portions

Makes approximately 16 ounces

Preparation time

15 minutes

Cooking time

No cooking required

Ingredients:

- 1/2 cup dried elderberries
- 1/4 cup dried nettle leaves
- 2 cups boiling water
- 1/2 cup raw honey
- 1 lemon, juiced

Instructions:

1. Place the dried elderberries and nettle leaves in a large heatproof jar or bowl.

2. Pour 2 cups of boiling water over the elderberries and nettle leaves.

3. Cover and allow the mixture to steep for at least 4 hours, or overnight for a stronger infusion.

4. Strain the mixture through a fine mesh strainer or cheesecloth, pressing to extract as much liquid as possible. Discard the solids.

5. Stir in the raw honey and lemon juice until well combined.

6. Transfer the tonic to a clean glass bottle or jar and seal tightly.

Variations:

- For added flavor and health benefits, infuse the tonic with a piece of ginger or a few sprigs of thyme while it steeps.

- Substitute honey with maple syrup for a vegan-friendly version.

Storage tips:

Store the Elderberry and Nettle Tonic in the refrigerator for up to 2 weeks. Shake well before each use.

Tips for allergens:

For those with allergies to honey, maple syrup serves as a suitable alternative that maintains the tonic's beneficial properties. Individuals with sensitivities to elderberry or nettle should consult with a healthcare provider before consuming this tonic.

97. Ginger and Lemon Tonic

Beneficial effects:

Ginger and Lemon Tonic is a refreshing and potent remedy designed to boost the immune system, aid digestion, and reduce inflammation. Ginger, with its powerful anti-inflammatory and antioxidant properties, helps to soothe sore throats, reduce nausea, and combat flu and cold symptoms. Lemon, rich in vitamin C, enhances the immune system, aids in detoxification, and provides a refreshing taste. This tonic is an excellent preventative measure to maintain overall health and well-being.

Ingredients:

- 1 tablespoon of freshly grated ginger
- Juice of 1 lemon
- 1 teaspoon of raw honey (optional, for sweetness)
- 2 cups of boiling water

Instructions:

1. Place the freshly grated ginger in a teapot or heatproof pitcher.

2. Add the juice of 1 lemon to the grated ginger.

3. Pour 2 cups of boiling water over the ginger and lemon juice.

4. Allow the mixture to steep for about 10 minutes.

5. Strain the tonic into a mug or glass to remove the ginger pieces.

6. Stir in 1 teaspoon of raw honey, if desired, until dissolved.

7. Enjoy the tonic warm or allow it to cool and serve over ice for a refreshing drink.

Variations:

- For an extra immune boost, add a pinch of cayenne pepper or turmeric to the tonic during the steeping process.
- Substitute honey with maple syrup for a vegan version or omit sweeteners entirely to enjoy the natural flavors.
- Add a sprig of mint or a slice of cucumber for a refreshing twist.

Storage tips:

The Ginger and Lemon Tonic is best enjoyed fresh. However, if you need to store it, keep it in the refrigerator in a sealed container for up to 24 hours. Reheat gently on the stove or enjoy cold.

Tips for allergens:

Individuals with sensitivities to citrus or ginger should adjust the amounts according to their tolerance or consult with a healthcare provider before consuming. For those avoiding honey due to allergies or dietary preferences, maple syrup or agave nectar are suitable alternatives that do not compromise the tonic's effectiveness.

98. Turmeric and Honey Tonic

Beneficial effects:

Turmeric and Honey Tonic is a powerful natural remedy designed to boost the immune system, reduce inflammation, and improve digestion. The curcumin in turmeric provides potent anti-inflammatory and antioxidant benefits, while honey adds antimicrobial properties and soothes the throat, making this tonic ideal for cold and flu prevention as well as overall health maintenance.

Ingredients:

- 1 teaspoon of turmeric powder
- 1 tablespoon of raw, organic honey
- 1 cup of warm water
- A pinch of black pepper (to enhance the absorption of curcumin)
- 1 teaspoon of lemon juice (optional, for added vitamin C and flavor)

Instructions:

1. Warm 1 cup of water to a comfortable drinking temperature.
2. Add 1 teaspoon of turmeric powder and a pinch of black pepper to the warm water.
3. Stir in 1 tablespoon of raw, organic honey until it is completely dissolved.
4. If desired, add 1 teaspoon of lemon juice for additional flavor and vitamin C.
5. Consume the tonic immediately, preferably on an empty stomach in the morning to maximize its health benefits.

Variations:

- For an extra immune boost, add a small piece of grated ginger to the tonic.

- To make a larger batch, multiply the ingredients accordingly and store in the refrigerator. Consume within 24 hours for best results.

Storage tips:

This tonic is best prepared fresh to ensure the maximum potency of its ingredients. However, if you need to prepare it in advance, store it in a tightly sealed glass container in the refrigerator and consume within 24 hours for best taste and benefits.

Tips for allergens:

Individuals with allergies to pollen or bee products should substitute honey with maple syrup or agave nectar to avoid any allergic reactions. Those with a sensitivity to turmeric or black pepper should start with a smaller dose to ensure tolerance.

99. Rosemary and Sage Tonic

Beneficial effects:

Rosemary and Sage Tonic is a refreshing and health-boosting drink that harnesses the natural powers of rosemary and sage, both of which are renowned for their anti-inflammatory, antioxidant, and antimicrobial properties. This tonic can help improve digestion, boost cognitive function, and support the immune system, making it an excellent addition to a daily wellness routine.

Ingredients:

- 1 tablespoon of fresh rosemary leaves
- 1 tablespoon of fresh sage leaves
- 2 cups of boiling water

- Honey or lemon to taste (optional)

Instructions:

1. Place the fresh rosemary and sage leaves in a heat-resistant pitcher or teapot.

2. Pour 2 cups of boiling water over the herbs.

3. Cover and allow the mixture to steep for 10 to 15 minutes.

4. Strain the tonic to remove the leaves.

5. If desired, add honey or lemon to taste.

6. Serve the tonic warm, or allow it to cool and enjoy it chilled.

Variations:

- For a cold-weather version, add a cinnamon stick and a slice of fresh ginger to the boiling water for added warmth and immune support.

- To make a refreshing summer drink, add slices of cucumber and a few sprigs of mint to the cooled tonic and refrigerate before serving.

Storage tips:

The tonic can be stored in the refrigerator for up to 2 days. Keep it in a sealed glass container to maintain freshness. If you prefer to enjoy the tonic warm, gently reheat it on the stove, but do not boil.

Tips for allergens:

Individuals with sensitivities to specific herbs should substitute rosemary and sage with other non-allergenic herbs such as thyme or lemon balm. If using honey as a sweetener, it can be replaced with maple syrup for those with allergies to bee products.

100. Hibiscus and Mint Tonic

Beneficial effects:

Hibiscus and Mint Tonic is a refreshing and health-boosting drink that combines the antioxidant properties of hibiscus with the soothing qualities of mint. This tonic is ideal for supporting the immune system, promoting hydration, and offering a natural way to reduce stress and anxiety. Hibiscus is known for its high vitamin C content and ability to lower blood pressure, while mint aids digestion and provides a calming effect.

Ingredients:

- 2 tablespoons of dried hibiscus flowers
- 1/4 cup of fresh mint leaves
- 4 cups of boiling water
- Honey or lemon to taste (optional)
- Ice cubes for serving

Instructions:

1. Place the dried hibiscus flowers and fresh mint leaves in a large pitcher.

2. Pour 4 cups of boiling water over the hibiscus and mint.

3. Allow the mixture to steep for 15-20 minutes.

4. Strain the tonic to remove the hibiscus flowers and mint leaves, transferring the liquid back into the pitcher.

5. If desired, add honey or lemon to taste, and stir well until fully dissolved.

6. Refrigerate the tonic until it is chilled.

7. Serve over ice cubes for a refreshing drink.

Variations:

- For a sparkling version, mix the chilled tonic with an equal part of sparkling water before serving.
- Add slices of cucumber or citrus fruits such as orange, lime, or lemon to the pitcher for added flavor and nutrients.
- Incorporate a stick of cinnamon or a few slices of ginger during the steeping process for a warm, spicy undertone.

Storage tips:

The Hibiscus and Mint Tonic can be stored in the refrigerator for up to 3 days. Keep it in a sealed pitcher or bottle to maintain freshness and prevent absorption of other flavors from the fridge.

Tips for allergens:

For those with allergies to pollen or specific herbs, ensure that both hibiscus and mint are suitable for your consumption. Honey can be substituted with maple syrup or agave nectar for those with allergies to bee products or for a vegan alternative.

Part V: Special Considerations

Herbs for Specific Populations

When considering herbal remedies, it's crucial to recognize that different life stages and conditions require tailored approaches. For instance, children, pregnant women, and the elderly have unique physiological needs and sensitivities. Likewise, individuals managing chronic conditions or those on multiple medications must proceed with caution. This section delves into these special considerations, offering guidance to safely incorporate herbal remedies into care for these specific populations.

Children's Health: The delicate systems of children respond well to gentle herbs such as chamomile for calming and sleep, echinacea for immune support, and fennel for digestive discomfort. However, dosages should be significantly reduced compared to adult amounts. A general guideline is to adjust the dose according to the child's age or weight, consulting a healthcare professional experienced in pediatric herbal medicine for precise recommendations.

Women's Health: Herbal remedies can play a supportive role in addressing women's health issues, from menstrual cramps and PMS to menopausal symptoms. Raspberry leaf tea, for example, is renowned for its benefits during pregnancy, while vitex (chaste tree berry) can help regulate menstrual cycles. However, due to the potential for herbs to affect hormonal balance, it's advisable to consult with a healthcare provider knowledgeable in herbal medicine before beginning any new regimen, especially during pregnancy and breastfeeding.

Elderly Care: As we age, metabolism and organ function can slow, affecting how the body processes medications, including herbal remedies. Elderly individuals also often manage multiple health conditions and medications, raising the risk of interactions. Therefore, starting with low doses and monitoring closely for any adverse effects is essential. Herbs like ginger can aid digestion and reduce inflammation, while ginkgo biloba may support cognitive function, but always under professional guidance to avoid contraindications.

Detoxification and Cleansing: While the body naturally detoxifies through the liver, kidneys, and other organs, certain herbs can support these processes. Milk thistle, for example, is well-regarded for its liver-protective properties. However, embarking on a detox regimen should be approached with caution, especially for those with underlying health conditions or those taking medications. Consulting with a healthcare professional can ensure that any detox plan is safe and effective.

Herbal First Aid: For minor cuts, burns, and bites, herbal remedies can provide immediate, on-the-spot care. Aloe vera gel soothes burns, while calendula cream can promote healing of cuts and scrapes. Having a herbal first aid kit prepared with these and other remedies like lavender essential oil for relaxation and tea tree oil for its antimicrobial properties can be invaluable. However, it's important to recognize the limits of self-care and seek professional medical attention for serious injuries or infections.

Incorporating herbs into daily life for specific populations or conditions requires careful consideration of the individual's overall health, existing medications, and the specific properties of the herbs. By doing so, herbal remedies can offer a complementary approach to enhancing well-being and addressing health challenges, all while minimizing risks and ensuring safety.

Herbs for Specific Populations

Addressing the unique needs of different populations is a pivotal aspect of herbal remedy application. Each group, be it children, women, the elderly, or those with specific health conditions, requires a nuanced approach to ensure both efficacy and safety. This segment focuses on guiding beginners through the process of selecting and using herbal remedies tailored to these specific demographics, emphasizing the importance of gentle, informed, and cautious application.

Children's Health: For young ones, the focus is on mild herbs and reduced dosages. Introducing herbs like chamomile, known for its soothing properties, can aid in sleep and calmness. Likewise, echinacea can be used to bolster the immune system during cold and flu season. It's crucial to consult with a pediatric healthcare provider familiar with herbal remedies to determine appropriate dosages based on the child's age and weight.

Women's Health: Women can benefit significantly from herbs that support hormonal balance and reproductive health. Raspberry leaf tea is a time-honored remedy for pregnancy support, known to tone the uterine muscles. Vitex, or chaste tree berry, is another herb that can help regulate menstrual cycles and alleviate symptoms of PMS. However, due to the profound effects herbs can have on hormonal balance, consultation with a healthcare provider is essential, especially during pregnancy and breastfeeding.

Elderly Care: As metabolism and organ function slow with age, the elderly population requires special consideration when using herbal remedies. Starting with lower doses and closely monitoring for any adverse effects is key. Herbs such as ginger can aid digestion and reduce inflammation, while ginkgo biloba supports cognitive function. Professional guidance is crucial to avoid interactions with medications and to tailor remedies to the individual's health profile.

Detoxification and Cleansing: Certain herbs support the body's natural detoxification processes, such as milk thistle for liver health. However, embarking on a detox or cleanse should be approached with caution, particularly for those with underlying health conditions or those taking prescription medications. A healthcare professional can provide guidance on safe and effective detoxification practices.

Herbal First Aid: For minor injuries and ailments, a well-prepared herbal first aid kit can be invaluable. Aloe vera gel for burns, calendula cream for cuts, and lavender essential oil for relaxation are just a few examples of herbal remedies that can provide immediate, natural care. Recognizing the limits of self-care and when to seek professional medical attention is essential for serious injuries or infections.

Incorporating herbal remedies into care for specific populations requires an understanding of the unique needs and sensitivities of each group. By doing so, herbal remedies can offer a complementary approach to enhancing well-being and addressing health challenges, all while minimizing risks and ensuring safety. Always consult with a healthcare professional before introducing new herbal remedies, especially for children, pregnant or breastfeeding women, the elderly, and those with chronic health conditions or taking multiple medications. This cautious, informed approach ensures that herbal remedies are used safely and effectively to support health and wellness across all stages of life.

Children's Health

Caring for children's health with herbal remedies requires a gentle and informed approach, recognizing the unique sensitivities and needs of their developing bodies. Herbal treatments can be a wonderful addition to a child's healthcare regimen, offering natural ways to support their immune system, soothe digestive disturbances, and promote relaxation and sleep. However, it's crucial to proceed with caution, ensuring that any herb introduced is safe for pediatric use and administered in appropriate dosages.

Objective: To safely use herbal remedies to support children's health, addressing common ailments such as colds, digestive issues, and difficulty sleeping with gentle, child-friendly herbs.

Preparation:

- Identify the child's specific health need or ailment.

- Choose herbs known for their safety and efficacy in children, such as chamomile, lavender, and echinacea.

- Consult with a pediatric healthcare provider experienced in herbal medicine to confirm the suitability and dosage of chosen herbs.

Materials:

- Dried or fresh chamomile flowers

- Dried or fresh lavender buds

- Echinacea root or flowers

- Clean, boiled water for teas

- Small glass jars with lids for storing any prepared remedies

Tools:

- Teapot or saucepan for brewing teas

- Fine mesh strainer or cheesecloth for straining teas

- Measuring spoons for precise dosing

Safety measures:

- Ensure all herbs are organic and sourced from reputable suppliers to avoid contaminants.

- Perform a patch test on the skin for any topical application to check for allergic reactions.

- Start with the lowest possible dose and observe the child for any adverse reactions.

Step-by-step Instructions:

1. **Chamomile Tea for Relaxation and Digestive Comfort**:

- Boil 1 cup of water.

- Add 1 teaspoon of dried chamomile flowers to the boiling water (half the adult dose).

- Steep for 5 minutes, then strain.

- Allow the tea to cool to a safe temperature before giving it to the child.

- **Dosage:** Give 1/4 to 1/2 cup of tea to the child, depending on age and size, up to twice a day.

2. **Lavender Infused Oil for Relaxation and Minor Skin Irritations**:

- Fill a small jar with dried lavender buds.

- Cover the buds with a carrier oil such as almond or coconut oil.

- Seal the jar and let it sit in a warm, sunny spot for 3-4 weeks, shaking daily.

- Strain the oil through cheesecloth into a clean jar.

- **Dosage:** Apply a small amount to the temples or back of the neck at bedtime for relaxation, or to minor cuts and scrapes as needed.

3. **Echinacea Tincture for Immune Support**:

- Consult with a healthcare provider for the appropriate dosage and ensure the child has no allergies to echinacea.

- Purchase a child-safe echinacea tincture from a reputable supplier, or make your own following safe home-tincture methods, ensuring the alcohol is fully evaporated before administration to remove alcohol content.

- **Dosage:** Typically, a very small amount diluted in water or juice, as directed by a healthcare provider, not exceeding twice a day during illness.

Cost estimate: Costs vary depending on the herbs and materials used but generally range from $5 to $20 for starting supplies.

Time estimate:

- Teas are ready in about 10-15 minutes.

- Infused oils and tinctures require several weeks for preparation but offer a longer shelf life.

Safety tips:

- Always supervise children when they are consuming herbal remedies.

- Keep all herbal remedies out of reach of children to prevent accidental ingestion.

Troubleshooting:

- If a child refuses to take a remedy due to taste, try diluting it further or mixing it with a small amount of their favorite juice.

- If skin irritation occurs with topical applications, discontinue use immediately and wash the area with soap and water.

Maintenance:

- Store dried herbs in a cool, dark place to preserve their potency.

- Keep prepared teas, oils, and tinctures in labeled, sealed containers, and use within the recommended timeframe.

Difficulty rating: ★☆☆☆☆ to ★★☆☆☆, depending on the remedy.

Variations:

- Combine chamomile and lavender in a tea to enhance relaxation effects.

- Add a small amount of honey to sweeten teas for children over 1 year old, if desired and not contraindicated.

By incorporating these gentle herbal remedies into a child's care routine, parents can naturally address common ailments, promoting comfort and well-being. Always prioritize safety by consulting healthcare professionals and closely observing the child's response to any new remedy.

Women's Health

Women's health encompasses a broad spectrum of concerns, from menstrual and reproductive issues to hormonal balance and menopausal support. Herbal remedies offer a natural pathway to address these concerns, providing relief and support without the harsh side effects often associated with conventional treatments. The key is to understand which herbs are beneficial for specific women's health issues and how to use them safely and effectively.

For menstrual cramps and PMS, herbs like cramp bark and black cohosh can offer significant relief. Cramp bark, as its name suggests, is particularly effective in alleviating menstrual cramps, thanks to its antispasmodic properties. To prepare a cramp bark tea, simmer one teaspoon of the dried bark in a cup of water for 10-15 minutes. Drink this tea two to three times a day during the menstrual period to ease cramps. Black cohosh, another powerful herb, has been traditionally used to treat not only menstrual cramps but also symptoms of menopause.

When it comes to fertility and reproductive health, red raspberry leaf is a powerhouse. Rich in vitamins and minerals, it is known to strengthen the uterine walls and may improve fertility outcomes. A simple way to incorporate red raspberry leaf is by drinking it as a tea. Steep one tablespoon of dried leaves in hot water for at least 15 minutes and drink one to three cups daily. It's not only beneficial for those trying to conceive but can also support uterine health throughout pregnancy.

For women navigating the challenges of menopause, sage and black cohosh offer comfort. Sage tea can help reduce night sweats and hot flashes, common symptoms of menopause. Brew by steeping one to two teaspoons of dried sage leaves in hot water for about 10 minutes. Drinking one cup daily can provide relief. Black cohosh, taken in capsule or tincture form, can also alleviate menopausal symptoms by mimicking estrogen in the body, which may lessen the frequency and intensity of hot flashes.

It's important to approach herbal remedies with mindfulness, especially in women's health, as the body's hormonal balance is delicate. Consulting with a healthcare provider knowledgeable in both conventional and herbal medicine is advisable before starting any new herbal regimen, particularly for pregnant or breastfeeding women, or those with pre-existing health conditions.

Materials:

- Cramp bark (dried bark)
- Black cohosh (dried root or tincture)
- Red raspberry leaf (dried leaves)
- Sage (dried leaves)

Tools:

- Teapot or saucepan

- Strainer

- Measuring spoons

- Cup or mug for serving

Safety measures:

- Always source herbs from reputable suppliers to ensure purity and safety.

- Start with small doses to monitor the body's response.

- Consult with a healthcare provider before beginning any new herbal treatment, especially if pregnant, breastfeeding, or managing a health condition.

Step-by-step Instructions: for preparing a basic herbal tea:

1. Measure the appropriate amount of dried herb (usually 1-2 teaspoons) per cup of water.

2. Boil water and pour over the herbs in a teapot or cup.

3. Cover and steep for the recommended time, usually 10-15 minutes.

4. Strain the tea and enjoy. Sweeten with honey if desired, but note that some herbs may have a naturally pleasant taste.

Cost estimate: Varies depending on the herb but generally ranges from $5 to $20 for enough herbs to last several months.

Time estimate: Preparation time is typically around 15-20 minutes, including boiling water and steeping.

Safety tips:

- Discontinue use if adverse reactions occur and consult a healthcare professional.

- Be cautious with dosages; more is not always better.

Troubleshooting:

- If the tea tastes too strong, dilute it with more water or reduce the steeping time.

- If no relief is observed after a few weeks, consult with a healthcare provider for further guidance.

Difficulty rating: ★☆☆☆☆. Preparing and using herbal remedies for women's health is straightforward and accessible for beginners.

By incorporating these herbal remedies into their wellness routines, women can harness the power of nature to support their health through every stage of life, from menstruation to menopause. Empowering oneself with knowledge about these natural solutions can lead to a more balanced, healthy life.

Elderly care in the realm of herbal remedies requires a nuanced understanding of how aging bodies respond to natural treatments. With metabolism slowing down and the possibility of multiple health conditions being managed simultaneously, the elderly population benefits from a careful, individualized approach to herbal supplementation. Herbs such as ginger, known for its digestive and anti-inflammatory properties, can be beneficial but must be introduced in smaller doses. Similarly, ginkgo biloba, which supports cognitive function and circulation, offers promise for enhancing the quality of life among seniors, yet it's crucial to monitor for interactions with prescription medications.

For those managing arthritis or joint pain, turmeric's curcumin content provides anti-inflammatory benefits. Incorporating turmeric into the diet or as a supplement needs to be balanced with an understanding of its blood-thinning effects, particularly for those on anticoagulant therapy. A simple preparation could involve adding turmeric to meals or preparing a golden milk beverage with a teaspoon of turmeric powder, a cup of warm milk (or a dairy-free alternative), a dash of black pepper to enhance curcumin absorption, and a teaspoon of honey for taste.

Sleep disturbances, a common issue among the elderly, may be alleviated with herbs like chamomile and lavender. A nightly cup of chamomile tea or using lavender essential oil in a diffuser can promote relaxation and improve sleep quality. However, it's essential to ensure that these remedies do not interfere with sleep medications.

Herbal remedies also offer support for heart health and circulation, with hawthorn being a standout for its cardiovascular benefits. Hawthorn can be taken as a tea or tincture, but starting with low doses under professional guidance is key to avoiding potential interactions with cardiac medications.

When introducing any new herb to an elderly individual's regimen, the following steps are recommended:

1. **Consultation with a Healthcare Provider**: Before starting any herbal remedy, consult with a healthcare professional, ideally one knowledgeable in both conventional and herbal medicine. This step is crucial to prevent adverse interactions with existing medications and conditions.

2. **Starting with Low Doses**: Begin with smaller doses than what might be used for younger adults. Observe the effects and adjust as necessary, always under professional supervision.

3. **Monitoring for Side Effects**: Keep a close watch for any new symptoms or changes in health that could indicate an adverse reaction to the herb. If any concerns arise, discontinue use and consult a healthcare provider.

4. **Quality and Purity of Herbs**: Source herbs from reputable suppliers to ensure they are free from contaminants and accurately labeled.

5. **Regular Review of Herbal Regimen**: As health conditions and medications change, regularly review the herbal regimen with a healthcare provider to ensure ongoing safety and efficacy.

Materials:

- Ginger root (fresh or dried for teas)

- Ginkgo biloba leaves (for teas or capsules)

- Turmeric powder

- Chamomile flowers (for tea)

- Lavender essential oil

- Hawthorn berries or leaves (for tea or tincture)

Tools:

- Teapot or saucepan for brewing teas

- Tea strainer

- Diffuser for essential oils

Safety measures:

- Always start with low doses

- Monitor for interactions with medications

- Consult with a healthcare provider before starting any new herbal remedy

By integrating these practices into the care plan for the elderly, herbal remedies can provide gentle, natural support for various health concerns, enhancing well-being while minimizing risks.

101. Milk Thistle Detox Tea

Beneficial effects:

Milk Thistle Detox Tea is a natural remedy designed to support liver health and promote detoxification. Milk thistle contains silymarin, a group of compounds known to have antioxidant, antiviral, and anti-inflammatory properties, making it beneficial for cleansing the liver, improving bile flow, and aiding in the digestion of fats. Regular consumption of this tea can help protect the liver from toxins, promote liver regeneration, and enhance overall detoxification processes.

Ingredients:

- 1 tablespoon of dried milk thistle seeds
- 2 cups of water
- Honey or lemon to taste (optional)

Instructions:

1. Crush the dried milk thistle seeds using a mortar and pestle to release their beneficial oils.

2. Bring 2 cups of water to a boil in a small saucepan.

3. Add the crushed milk thistle seeds to the boiling water.

4. Reduce the heat and simmer for 20 minutes.

5. Remove from heat and allow the tea to steep for an additional 20 minutes.

6. Strain the tea into a cup or mug, removing the milk thistle seeds.

7. If desired, add honey or lemon to taste.

8. Enjoy the tea warm, preferably in the morning before breakfast or in the evening before bedtime.

Variations:

- For added detoxification benefits, include a teaspoon of dandelion root or ginger in the tea while simmering.

- To create a blend for enhanced liver support, mix milk thistle seeds with turmeric and green tea leaves during the simmering process.

Storage tips:

Store leftover dried milk thistle seeds in an airtight container in a cool, dark place to maintain their potency. Prepared milk thistle detox tea can be refrigerated in a sealed container for up to 48 hours. Reheat gently without boiling before consuming.

Tips for allergens:

Individuals with allergies to plants in the Asteraceae family, such as daisies, marigolds, or chrysanthemums, should proceed with caution when consuming milk thistle tea. If using honey as a sweetener, those with allergies to bee products can substitute it with maple syrup or enjoy the tea without sweeteners.

102. Dandelion and Burdock Root Cleanse

Beneficial effects:

The Dandelion and Burdock Root Cleanse is designed to support the body's natural detoxification processes, promoting liver health and aiding in the removal of toxins from the bloodstream. Dandelion root acts as a powerful diuretic, increasing urine production to help flush out waste, while burdock root is rich in antioxidants that can protect liver cells from damage and stimulate bile production to aid in digestion.

Ingredients:

- 1 tablespoon of dried dandelion root
- 1 tablespoon of dried burdock root
- 4 cups of water
- Lemon slices or honey (optional, for flavor)

Instructions:

1. Combine the dried dandelion root and dried burdock root in a medium-sized pot.

2. Add 4 cups of water to the pot and bring the mixture to a boil.

3. Once boiling, reduce the heat and let the mixture simmer for about 15 minutes.

4. After simmering, remove the pot from the heat and allow the mixture to steep for an additional 15 minutes to enhance the extraction of beneficial compounds.

5. Strain the mixture into a large pitcher or jar, discarding the solid root pieces.

6. If desired, add lemon slices or a teaspoon of honey to the warm mixture for added flavor.

7. Consume 1 cup of the cleanse tea in the morning on an empty stomach and another cup in the evening before dinner.

Variations:

- For a cold beverage option, allow the tea to cool to room temperature, then refrigerate for 1-2 hours. Serve over ice if desired.
- Add a slice of fresh ginger during the simmering process for an additional detoxifying effect and a spicy flavor.

Storage tips:

The Dandelion and Burdock Root Cleanse can be stored in the refrigerator for up to 48 hours. Keep it in a sealed glass container to maintain freshness. It's best to prepare a fresh batch every two days to ensure potency.

Tips for allergens:

Individuals with allergies to dandelion, burdock, or related plants should consult with a healthcare provider before starting this cleanse. For those with sensitivities to honey, maple syrup can be used as a sweetener alternative.

103. Parsley and Cilantro Detox Smoothie

Beneficial effects:

The Parsley and Cilantro Detox Smoothie is a potent detoxifying blend that supports the body's natural detoxification processes, particularly in the liver and kidneys. Parsley is rich in vitamins A, C, and K, and has diuretic properties that can help eliminate toxins. Cilantro, on the other hand, has been shown to bind to heavy metals, facilitating their removal from the body. Together, these herbs create a powerful detox smoothie that not only aids in cleansing but also provides a boost of essential nutrients.

Portions

Serves 2

Preparation time

10 minutes

Ingredients:

- 1 cup of fresh parsley leaves
- 1 cup of fresh cilantro leaves
- 1 ripe banana
- 1/2 cup of pineapple chunks
- 1 tablespoon of fresh lemon juice
- 1 teaspoon of grated ginger
- 1 cup of coconut water
- Ice cubes (optional)

Instructions:

1. Wash the parsley and cilantro leaves thoroughly to remove any dirt or residue.
2. Place the parsley, cilantro, banana, pineapple, lemon juice, and grated ginger into a blender.
3. Add the coconut water to the blender. If you prefer a colder smoothie, add a few ice cubes as well.
4. Blend on high until the mixture is smooth and creamy.
5. Taste the smoothie and adjust the sweetness or acidity as needed by adding more pineapple or lemon juice.
6. Pour the smoothie into two glasses and serve immediately for the best flavor and nutrient content.

Variations:

- For an extra detoxifying boost, add a tablespoon of chia seeds or flaxseeds to the blender before mixing.
- If you prefer a sweeter smoothie, add a tablespoon of honey or agave syrup.
- To increase the smoothie's fiber content, include a handful of spinach or kale.

Storage tips:

This detox smoothie is best enjoyed fresh. However, if you need to store it, keep it in an airtight container in the refrigerator for up to 24 hours. Give it a good stir or shake before drinking, as separation may occur.

Tips for allergens:

For those with allergies to citrus, you can omit the lemon juice and substitute it with a teaspoon of apple cider vinegar for a similar detoxifying effect. If you're allergic to pineapple, consider replacing it with mango or peaches to maintain the smoothie's sweetness and texture.

104. Lemon and Ginger Detox Water

Beneficial effects:

Lemon and Ginger Detox Water is a refreshing and powerful detoxifying drink that aids in digestion, boosts the immune system, and helps to cleanse the liver. The combination of lemon and ginger works synergistically to flush out toxins, reduce inflammation, and provide a rich source of antioxidants. This detox water is perfect for starting your day or enjoying as a revitalizing beverage anytime.

Ingredients:

- 1/2 lemon, thinly sliced
- 1-inch piece of ginger, thinly sliced
- 4 cups of water
- Ice cubes (optional)

Instructions:

1. Place the lemon slices and ginger slices in a large pitcher.

2. Add 4 cups of water to the pitcher.

3. Refrigerate the mixture for at least 1 hour to allow the flavors to infuse. Overnight is best for maximum benefits.

4. Serve the detox water over ice cubes if desired.

Variations:

- Add a few sprigs of fresh mint or a teaspoon of honey for additional flavor and health benefits.

- For a sparkling version, replace 1 cup of water with sparkling water just before serving.

- Incorporate cucumber slices for an extra detoxifying effect and refreshing taste.

Storage tips:

This detox water can be stored in the refrigerator for up to 24 hours. For best taste, consume within this time frame as the lemon and ginger may start to become bitter if left to infuse for too long.

Tips for allergens:

For those with sensitivities to citrus, the lemon can be replaced with cucumber or omitted entirely. If ginger is a concern, it can be reduced or removed without significantly altering the detoxifying benefits of the drink.

105. Activated Charcoal Lemonade

Beneficial effects:

Activated Charcoal Lemonade is a detoxifying drink that harnesses the powerful cleansing properties of activated charcoal, known for its ability to bind to toxins and chemicals, aiding in their removal from the body. This lemonade not only supports the body's natural detoxification processes but also helps in improving digestion and boosting energy levels. The addition of lemon enhances the detox effect with its high vitamin C content and aids in alkalizing the body, promoting overall well-being.

Ingredients:

- 2 tablespoons of activated charcoal powder (from coconut shells)
- Juice of 3 lemons
- 2 tablespoons of raw honey or maple syrup
- 4 cups of water
- Ice cubes (optional)

- A pinch of Himalayan pink salt (for electrolytes and minerals)

Instructions:

1. In a large pitcher, combine the lemon juice, raw honey or maple syrup, and water. Stir well until the honey or syrup is completely dissolved.

2. Add the activated charcoal powder to the pitcher. Stir thoroughly until the charcoal is fully incorporated into the liquid.

3. Add a pinch of Himalayan pink salt and stir.

4. Serve the lemonade over ice cubes if desired.

Variations:

- For a sparkling version, replace 2 cups of water with sparkling water, adding it to the pitcher just before serving to maintain its fizz.

- Add a few sprigs of fresh mint or a slice of ginger for additional flavor and digestive benefits.

Storage tips:

This lemonade is best enjoyed fresh. However, if you have leftovers, store them in a sealed glass container in the refrigerator for up to 24 hours. Shake well before serving as the activated charcoal may settle to the bottom.

Tips for allergens:

If you have allergies to bee products, substitute raw honey with maple syrup. Always ensure that the activated charcoal used is suitable for consumption and free from any additives that could cause allergic reactions.

106. Green Detox Soup

Beneficial effects:

Green Detox Soup is crafted to support detoxification and cleansing, offering a nourishing blend of vegetables and herbs known for their purifying properties. This soup aids in flushing out toxins, stimulating digestion, and replenishing the body with essential nutrients and antioxidants. It's an ideal choice for those looking to reset their digestive system, boost immune function, and promote overall health and vitality.

Portions

Serves 4

Preparation time

20 minutes

Cooking time

30 minutes

Ingredients:

- 4 cups of vegetable broth
- 2 cups of water
- 1 cup of chopped kale
- 1 cup of broccoli florets
- 1/2 cup of diced celery
- 1/2 cup of sliced carrots
- 1/2 cup of chopped parsley
- 1/4 cup of chopped cilantro
- 2 tablespoons of olive oil
- 1 medium onion, diced
- 2 cloves of garlic, minced
- 1 inch of fresh ginger, grated
- Juice of 1 lemon
- Salt and pepper to taste

Instructions:

1. Heat the olive oil in a large pot over medium heat.

2. Add the diced onion, minced garlic, and grated ginger to the pot. Sauté for 5 minutes, or until the onions are translucent.

3. Add the chopped kale, broccoli florets, diced celery, and sliced carrots to the pot. Stir well to combine.

4. Pour in the vegetable broth and water. Bring the mixture to a boil.

5. Reduce the heat to low and simmer for 20 minutes, or until the vegetables are tender.

6. Stir in the chopped parsley, cilantro, and lemon juice. Season with salt and pepper to taste.

7. Simmer for an additional 5 minutes.

8. Serve the soup warm.

Variations:

- For a spicy kick, add a pinch of cayenne pepper or a dash of hot sauce before serving.

- Incorporate other detoxifying ingredients such as spinach, dandelion greens, or turmeric for additional health benefits.

- For a creamier texture, blend half of the soup until smooth and then mix it back into the pot.

Storage tips:

Store any leftover Green Detox Soup in an airtight container in the refrigerator for up to 3 days. Reheat on the stove or in the microwave before serving. The soup can also be frozen for up to 1 month. Thaw in the refrigerator overnight and reheat thoroughly.

Tips for allergens:

For those with allergies to specific vegetables or herbs used in this recipe, feel free to substitute with other non-allergenic greens or herbs. Olive oil can be replaced with avocado oil for those with olive sensitivities.

107. Beetroot and Carrot Juice Cleanse

Beneficial effects:

The Beetroot and Carrot Juice Cleanse is designed to support detoxification and cleansing of the body. Rich in antioxidants, vitamins, and minerals, this juice can help improve liver function, aid in flushing out toxins, and promote healthy skin. Beetroot contains betalains, compounds that have been shown to provide antioxidant, anti-inflammatory, and detoxification support. Carrots are high in beta-carotene, which is converted into vitamin A in the body, supporting immune function and eye health. Together, these ingredients create a powerful detoxifying drink that can rejuvenate and energize the body.

Ingredients:

- 2 medium beetroots, peeled and chopped
- 4 large carrots, peeled and chopped
- 1 inch of fresh ginger root, peeled
- 1 lemon, peeled
- 1 apple (optional, for sweetness)
- 2 cups of water

Instructions:

1. Wash all the fruits and vegetables thoroughly under running water.

2. Peel the beetroots, carrots, and ginger root. Chop them into small pieces to fit into your juicer.

3. Peel the lemon, removing as much of the white pith as possible to avoid bitterness.

4. If you're adding an apple for sweetness, core it and cut into wedges.

5. Add all the ingredients into the juicer, starting with the softer ones like lemon and apple, followed by ginger, carrots, and beetroots.

6. Juice all the ingredients. If the mixture is too thick, add water to achieve your desired consistency.

7. Pour the juice through a strainer into a large glass or pitcher to remove any pulp.

8. Serve the juice immediately, or chill in the refrigerator for an hour before serving.

Variations:

- For a spicy kick, add a pinch of cayenne pepper to the juice before serving.

- Include a handful of leafy greens like spinach or kale for additional detoxification benefits.

- Substitute the apple with a pear for a different type of sweetness.

Storage tips:

This juice is best enjoyed fresh to maximize the benefits of the nutrients. However, if you need to store it, keep the juice in an airtight container in the refrigerator for up to 24 hours. Shake well before drinking, as separation is natural.

Tips for allergens:

For individuals with allergies to any of the ingredients listed, simply omit or substitute with another fruit or vegetable of your choice. For example, if allergic to apples, using a pear or adding more lemon can provide a pleasant alternative without compromising the detoxifying benefits of the juice.

108. Cucumber and Mint Detox Water

Beneficial effects:

Cucumber and Mint Detox Water is a refreshing and hydrating drink that aids in detoxification and cleansing of the body. Cucumbers are rich in antioxidants and help flush out toxins, while mint promotes digestion and adds a soothing flavor. This detox water is perfect for those looking to improve their hydration, support natural detox processes, and enhance overall health.

Portions

Serves 2

Preparation time

5 minutes

Ingredients:

- 1 medium cucumber, thinly sliced
- 10 fresh mint leaves
- 4 cups of water
- Ice cubes (optional)
- Lemon slices for garnish (optional)

Instructions:

1. In a large pitcher, combine the thinly sliced cucumber and fresh mint leaves.

2. Add 4 cups of water to the pitcher.

3. If desired, add ice cubes to the pitcher for an extra chill.

4. Stir the mixture gently to combine the flavors.

5. Let the detox water sit for at least 1 hour in the refrigerator to allow the flavors to infuse. For best results, let it infuse overnight.

6. Serve the detox water in glasses, garnished with lemon slices if desired.

Variations:

- For a sweeter taste, add a teaspoon of honey or agave syrup to the water before refrigerating.

- Include slices of ginger for an additional detoxifying effect and a spicy kick.

- Swap out mint for basil or rosemary for a different herbal note.

Storage tips:

The Cucumber and Mint Detox Water can be stored in the refrigerator for up to 24 hours. It's best to consume it within this time frame to enjoy its fresh taste and maximum benefits.

Tips for allergens:

This recipe is naturally allergen-free. However, for those with specific plant sensitivities, ensure that both cucumber and mint are suitable for your consumption. Lemon and additional ingredients like ginger or honey should also be used according to individual dietary tolerances and preferences.

109. Turmeric and Lemon Detox Drink

Beneficial effects:

The Turmeric and Lemon Detox Drink is a revitalizing beverage that harnesses the detoxifying powers of turmeric and the cleansing benefits of lemon. Turmeric, with its active compound curcumin, offers potent anti-inflammatory and antioxidant properties, aiding in the detoxification process and supporting liver health. Lemon, rich in vitamin C, enhances the immune system and promotes skin health while stimulating the digestive system to flush out toxins. This detox drink is ideal for those looking to naturally cleanse their body, boost their immune system, and improve overall vitality.

Ingredients:

- 1 teaspoon of turmeric powder
- Juice of 1 lemon
- 1 tablespoon of raw honey (optional, for sweetness)
- A pinch of black pepper (to enhance curcumin absorption)
- 2 cups of warm water

Instructions:

1. Warm 2 cups of water to a comfortable drinking temperature.

2. Add 1 teaspoon of turmeric powder and a pinch of black pepper to the warm water.

3. Squeeze the juice of 1 lemon into the mixture.

4. Stir in 1 tablespoon of raw honey, if desired, until fully dissolved.

5. Consume the drink warm, preferably in the morning on an empty stomach to maximize its detoxifying benefits.

Variations:

- For an added boost, include a teaspoon of grated ginger to the drink for its digestive and anti-inflammatory benefits.

- Replace warm water with green tea for an extra antioxidant kick.

- For those who prefer a cold beverage, allow the drink to cool and serve over ice.

Storage tips:

This detox drink is best consumed fresh to ensure the potency of its ingredients. However, if preparing in advance, store it in the refrigerator in a glass container for up to 24 hours. Shake well before consuming.

Tips for allergens:

Individuals with allergies to pollen or bee products should substitute honey with maple syrup or simply omit the sweetener. Those sensitive to turmeric or black pepper should adjust the quantities according to their tolerance or consult with a healthcare provider before incorporating this drink into their routine.

110. Apple and Cinnamon Detox Water

Beneficial effects:

Apple and Cinnamon Detox Water is a refreshing and health-enhancing beverage designed to support detoxification and cleansing. Apples provide essential vitamins, minerals, and antioxidants that promote health, while cinnamon offers anti-inflammatory properties and helps regulate blood sugar levels. This combination not only hydrates the body but also aids in flushing out toxins, improving digestion, and boosting the immune system.

Ingredients:

- 1 apple, thinly sliced
- 1 cinnamon stick
- 2 liters of water

Instructions:

1. Place the thinly sliced apple and cinnamon stick in a large pitcher.

2. Fill the pitcher with 2 liters of water.

3. Refrigerate the mixture for at least 1 hour to allow the flavors to infuse. For a stronger infusion, let it sit overnight.

4. Serve the detox water chilled. You can refill the pitcher with water a few times until the flavors begin to fade.

Variations:

- Add a few slices of fresh ginger for an additional detoxifying effect and a spicy kick.

- Include a handful of fresh mint leaves for a refreshing flavor and extra digestive benefits.

- For a sweeter taste, add a teaspoon of honey or a few drops of stevia to your glass before drinking.

Storage tips:

The Apple and Cinnamon Detox Water can be stored in the refrigerator for up to 3 days. Keep it in a sealed pitcher to maintain freshness and prevent any refrigerator odors from affecting the taste.

Tips for allergens:

For individuals with specific fruit allergies, the apple can be substituted with cucumber or citrus fruits like lemons and oranges, which also offer detoxifying benefits. If you have a sensitivity to cinnamon, simply omit it from the recipe or replace it with a few fresh basil leaves for a different flavor profile.

111. *Milk Thistle and Dandelion Detox Tea*

Beneficial effects:

Milk Thistle and Dandelion Detox Tea is a powerful combination aimed at supporting liver health and promoting the body's natural detoxification processes. Milk thistle is known for its liver-protecting properties, primarily due to silymarin, a group of compounds said to have antioxidant and anti-inflammatory effects. Dandelion root, on the other hand, acts as a diuretic, increasing urine output to help flush toxins from the body. Together, these herbs work synergistically to cleanse the liver, improve bile flow, and support overall detoxification.

Ingredients:

- 1 tablespoon of dried milk thistle seeds
- 1 tablespoon of dried dandelion root
- 4 cups of water
- Honey or lemon to taste (optional)

Instructions:

1. Crush the dried milk thistle seeds and dandelion root using a mortar and pestle to release their active ingredients.

2. Bring 4 cups of water to a boil in a medium-sized pot.

3. Add the crushed milk thistle seeds and dandelion root to the boiling water.

4. Reduce the heat and simmer for 15 minutes to allow the herbs to infuse their properties into the water.

5. Remove from heat and let the tea steep for an additional 10 minutes.

6. Strain the tea into a large pitcher or individual cups, discarding the used herbs.

7. If desired, add honey or lemon to taste.

8. Serve the tea warm, or allow it to cool and refrigerate for a refreshing cold drink.

Variations:

- For an added detox boost, include a slice of fresh ginger or a teaspoon of turmeric powder while simmering the tea.

- Mix in a handful of fresh mint leaves after removing the tea from heat for a refreshing flavor.

Storage tips:

This detox tea can be stored in the refrigerator for up to 48 hours. Ensure it's kept in an airtight container to maintain its freshness and potency. Reheat gently on the stove or enjoy cold.

Tips for allergens:

Individuals with allergies to plants in the Asteraceae family, such as daisies or ragweed, which includes dandelion, should proceed with caution and may want to consult with a healthcare provider before consuming this tea. For those avoiding honey due to allergies or dietary preferences, maple syrup can be used as a sweetener alternative.

112. Parsley and Lemon Detox Smoothie

Beneficial effects:

The Parsley and Lemon Detox Smoothie is a vibrant, nutrient-rich beverage designed to support the body's natural detoxification processes. Rich in antioxidants, vitamins, and minerals, parsley acts as a natural diuretic, helping to eliminate toxins and excess water from the body. Lemon, high in vitamin C, aids in cleansing the liver and improving digestion, making this smoothie an excellent choice for those looking to refresh and rejuvenate their system.

Portions

Serves 2

Preparation time

10 minutes

Ingredients:

- 1 cup fresh parsley leaves
- Juice of 2 lemons
- 1 cup cucumber, chopped
- 1 apple, cored and sliced
- 1 tablespoon chia seeds
- 2 cups water or coconut water
- Ice cubes (optional)

Instructions:

1. Wash the parsley leaves thoroughly to remove any dirt or residue.

2. In a blender, combine the parsley leaves, lemon juice, chopped cucumber, sliced apple, and chia seeds.

3. Add water or coconut water to the blender. For a chilled smoothie, add ice cubes as desired.

4. Blend on high until the mixture is smooth and creamy.

5. Taste the smoothie and adjust the sweetness or tartness by adding more apple or lemon juice if needed.

6. Pour the smoothie into glasses and serve immediately for maximum freshness and nutrient content.

Variations:

- For an extra boost of fiber and antioxidants, add a handful of spinach or kale to the smoothie before blending.

- If you prefer a sweeter smoothie, add a teaspoon of honey or agave syrup.

- To enhance the detoxifying effects, include a small piece of ginger or a pinch of turmeric powder.

Storage tips:

This detox smoothie is best enjoyed fresh. However, if you need to store it, keep it in an airtight container in the refrigerator for up to 24 hours. Stir well before serving as separation may occur.

Tips for allergens:

For those with allergies to citrus, you can omit the lemon juice and substitute it with a teaspoon of apple cider vinegar for a similar detoxifying effect. If allergic to chia seeds, they can be omitted or replaced with flaxseeds for a similar nutritional profile.

113. Cilantro and Ginger Detox Juice

Beneficial effects:

Cilantro and Ginger Detox Juice is a potent blend designed to cleanse the body, support digestion, and boost the immune system. Cilantro is known for its heavy metal detoxifying properties, while ginger aids in improving digestion and reducing inflammation. This juice is an excellent choice for those looking to naturally detoxify their body and enhance overall health.

Ingredients:

- 1 cup of fresh cilantro leaves
- 1 inch of fresh ginger, peeled and sliced
- Juice of 2 lemons
- 1 tablespoon of raw honey
- 2 cups of water

Instructions:

1. Wash the cilantro leaves thoroughly to remove any dirt or debris.
2. Peel and slice the ginger.
3. In a blender, combine the cilantro leaves, sliced ginger, lemon juice, raw honey, and water.
4. Blend on high until the mixture is smooth.
5. Strain the juice through a fine mesh sieve or cheesecloth into a pitcher, pressing to extract as much liquid as possible.
6. Serve the detox juice immediately, or chill in the refrigerator for an hour before serving.

Variations:

- For an extra immune boost, add a pinch of cayenne pepper to the juice before blending.
- If you prefer a sweeter juice, adjust the amount of honey according to your taste or substitute it with maple syrup for a vegan option.
- Add a cucumber to the blend for additional hydration and detoxifying benefits.

Storage tips:

This detox juice is best enjoyed fresh. However, if you have leftovers, store them in an airtight container in the refrigerator for up to 24 hours. Shake well before serving as natural separation may occur.

Tips for allergens:

Individuals with allergies to cilantro or ginger should omit these ingredients and consult with a healthcare provider for alternative detoxifying ingredients. For those with allergies to bee products, maple syrup can be used as a sweetener instead of honey.

114. Turmeric and Cucumber Detox Water

Beneficial effects:

Turmeric and Cucumber Detox Water is designed to hydrate and cleanse the body while providing anti-inflammatory benefits. Turmeric contains curcumin, a compound known for its antioxidant properties that can help reduce inflammation and boost the immune system. Cucumber aids in hydration and provides essential vitamins and minerals for overall health. This detox water is an excellent choice for those looking to support their body's natural detoxification processes, improve skin health, and enhance digestion.

Ingredients:

- 1/2 cucumber, thinly sliced
- 1 tablespoon of turmeric powder
- 1/2 lemon, thinly sliced
- 4 cups of water
- Ice cubes (optional)
- A pinch of black pepper (to enhance the absorption of curcumin)

Instructions:

1. In a large pitcher, combine the thinly sliced cucumber and lemon with the turmeric powder.

2. Add a pinch of black pepper to the mixture. This helps increase the bioavailability of curcumin in turmeric.

3. Fill the pitcher with 4 cups of water and stir well to combine all the ingredients.

4. If desired, add ice cubes to the pitcher for an extra chill.

5. Refrigerate the detox water for at least 1 hour to allow the flavors to infuse. Overnight infusion is recommended for stronger flavor and benefits.

6. Serve chilled, and enjoy the refreshing taste and detoxifying benefits of the water.

Variations:

- For a sweeter version, add a tablespoon of honey or maple syrup to the water before refrigerating.

- Include a few sprigs of fresh mint or a teaspoon of grated ginger for additional flavor and digestive benefits.

- Swap out lemon for lime for a different citrus twist.

Storage tips:

This detox water can be stored in the refrigerator for up to 24 hours. For best taste and benefits, consume within this time frame as the flavors may start to diminish beyond that.

Tips for allergens:

Individuals with allergies to cucumbers or citrus should substitute these ingredients with other fruits or vegetables, such as apples or celery, to avoid any allergic reactions. For those sensitive to black pepper, it can be omitted; however, this may reduce the bioavailability of curcumin from turmeric.

115. Beetroot and Lemon Detox Drink

Beneficial effects:

The Beetroot and Lemon Detox Drink is designed to support the body's natural detoxification processes, promoting liver health and aiding in the elimination of toxins. Beetroot is rich in antioxidants, vitamins, and minerals that help protect the liver and improve its function. Lemon, high in vitamin C, enhances the immune system and aids in digestion, further supporting the detox process. This drink is an excellent choice for those looking to cleanse their system, boost energy levels, and improve overall health.

Ingredients:

- 1 large beetroot, peeled and chopped
- Juice of 1 lemon
- 1 tablespoon of raw honey
- 2 cups of water
- Ice cubes (optional)

Instructions:

1. Place the chopped beetroot in a blender.

2. Add the lemon juice and raw honey.

3. Pour in 2 cups of water.

4. Blend on high until smooth.

5. Strain the mixture through a fine mesh sieve into a pitcher, pressing down to extract as much liquid as possible.

6. Discard the solids.

7. Serve the detox drink over ice cubes if desired, or chill in the refrigerator before serving.

Variations:

- For an added kick and to boost the detoxifying properties, include a piece of ginger or a pinch of cayenne pepper when blending.

- Substitute honey with maple syrup for a vegan option.

- Add a sprig of mint or a slice of cucumber for a refreshing twist.

Storage tips:

This detox drink is best enjoyed fresh. However, it can be stored in the refrigerator for up to 24 hours. Ensure it's kept in a sealed glass container to maintain freshness and prevent absorption of other flavors.

Tips for allergens:

Individuals with allergies to beets should avoid this drink. For those with sensitivities to citrus, the lemon juice can be reduced or omitted, adjusting the sweetness with additional honey or maple syrup as needed.

116. Comfrey Salve

Beneficial effects:

Comfrey Salve is renowned for its remarkable healing properties, particularly in the treatment of bruises, sprains, and minor burns. The active compound allantoin promotes cell regeneration, speeding up the healing process and reducing inflammation. This makes comfrey salve an essential component of any herbal first aid kit, offering a natural and effective solution for skin repair and relief from discomfort.

Ingredients:

- 1/4 cup dried comfrey leaves
- 1/2 cup olive oil
- 2 tablespoons beeswax
- 10 drops lavender essential oil (optional, for additional antiseptic and soothing properties)

Instructions:

1. In a double boiler, infuse the olive oil with dried comfrey leaves by gently heating them together for about 2-3 hours on low heat. Ensure the oil does not boil.

2. After infusion, strain the oil through a cheesecloth or fine mesh strainer to remove the comfrey leaves. Squeeze or press the leaves to extract as much oil as possible.

3. Return the infused oil to the double boiler and add the beeswax.

4. Heat gently, stirring constantly, until the beeswax is completely melted and mixed with the oil.

5. Remove from heat. If using, stir in the lavender essential oil.

6. Pour the mixture into small tins or jars. Let it cool and solidify at room temperature.

7. Once solidified, cover with lids and label the containers with the contents and date.

Variations:

- For a vegan version, substitute beeswax with an equal amount of candelilla wax or soy wax.

- Add vitamin E oil (a few drops) to the mixture before it solidifies for added skin healing benefits.

- Customize the salve with different essential oils based on your preferences or specific skin needs. Tea tree oil can be used for its antimicrobial properties, while chamomile oil can provide additional soothing effects.

Storage tips:

Store the comfrey salve in a cool, dark place. If stored properly, the salve can last for up to a year. Avoid exposing it to direct sunlight or heat, as this can cause the salve to melt.

Tips for allergens:

Individuals with sensitivities to comfrey or any of the essential oils should perform a patch test on a small area of skin before widespread application. If irritation occurs, discontinue use immediately. For those allergic to beeswax, using a plant-based wax alternative is recommended.

117. *Plantain Poultice*

Beneficial effects:

Plantain Poultice is a traditional remedy known for its soothing and healing properties, particularly effective in treating cuts, insect bites, and skin irritations. Plantain leaves contain allantoin, an anti-inflammatory compound that promotes wound healing, reduces pain, and stimulates the growth of new skin cells. This makes the poultice an excellent choice for natural first aid care, providing relief and accelerating recovery.

Ingredients:

- A handful of fresh plantain leaves
- Water (as needed)
- A clean cloth or gauze

Instructions:

1. Rinse the fresh plantain leaves thoroughly under running water to remove any dirt or debris.

2. Crush the leaves using a mortar and pestle or a rolling pin to release their juices. If necessary, add a few drops of water to help form a paste.

3. Spread the crushed plantain leaves directly onto the affected area of the skin. If the area is sensitive, place the leaves on a clean cloth or gauze first, then apply to the skin.

4. Secure the poultice in place with a bandage or another piece of cloth.

5. Leave the poultice on for up to 4 hours for adults or 2 hours for children. For sensitive skin, check the area frequently and remove if any irritation occurs.

6. After removal, gently wash the area with warm water and pat dry.

Variations:

- For added antimicrobial properties, mix the plantain leaves with a small amount of raw honey before applying.
- To enhance the poultice's soothing effect, add a few drops of lavender essential oil to the crushed plantain leaves.

Storage tips:

Fresh plantain leaves are best used immediately after picking. However, if you need to store them, wrap the leaves in a damp paper towel and place them in a plastic bag in the refrigerator for up to 2 days.

Tips for allergens:

Individuals with plant allergies should perform a patch test on a small area of skin before applying the poultice widely. If irritation or an allergic reaction occurs, discontinue use immediately.

118. Yarrow Powder

Beneficial effects:

Yarrow Powder is renowned for its ability to stop bleeding, making it an essential component of any herbal first aid kit. Its astringent and anti-inflammatory properties help in the quick clotting of blood and can prevent infections in cuts, scrapes, and deeper wounds. Yarrow is also known for its ability to reduce inflammation and promote healing, making it beneficial for treating bruises and swelling.

Ingredients:

- 1 part dried yarrow leaves and flowers
- Mortar and pestle or a spice grinder

Instructions:

1. Ensure the yarrow leaves and flowers are completely dried.

2. Place the dried yarrow in a mortar and pestle or a spice grinder.

3. Grind the yarrow until it forms a fine powder.

4. Store the yarrow powder in a clean, dry jar with a tightly fitting lid.

Variations:

- For an enhanced healing powder, mix equal parts of yarrow powder with powdered comfrey and plantain leaves. This combination creates a powerful herbal remedy that can be applied to wounds for faster healing.

- To make a yarrow-infused oil, which can be applied to wounds or used to create salves, fill a jar with dried yarrow and cover it with olive oil. Let it sit for 4-6 weeks, shaking occasionally, then strain and store in a clean jar.

Storage tips:

Store the yarrow powder in a cool, dark place. When stored properly, it can last for up to a year. Ensure the jar is tightly sealed to prevent moisture from entering, as this can cause the powder to clump or mold.

Tips for allergens:

Individuals with allergies to plants in the Asteraceae family, such as daisies, chrysanthemums, or ragweed, should proceed with caution when using yarrow. Always perform a patch test on a small area of skin before applying yarrow powder to wounds or bruises to ensure no allergic reaction occurs.

119. Calendula Ointment

Beneficial effects:

Calendula Ointment is renowned for its soothing, anti-inflammatory, and healing properties, making it an excellent remedy for treating minor cuts, scrapes, burns, and chapped skin. The active compounds in calendula, such as flavonoids and saponins, contribute to its ability to promote wound healing, reduce inflammation, and support skin health.

Ingredients:

- 1/4 cup dried calendula petals
- 1/2 cup olive oil
- 2 tablespoons beeswax pellets
- 1 teaspoon honey (optional, for added antimicrobial properties)
- 5 drops of lavender essential oil (optional, for fragrance and additional soothing effect)

Instructions:

1. Infuse the olive oil with dried calendula petals. Place the petals in a jar, cover with olive oil, seal the jar, and let it sit in a warm, sunny spot for 2-4 weeks. Shake the jar daily.

2. After the infusion period, strain the oil through a cheesecloth to remove the calendula petals.

3. In a double boiler, gently heat the infused olive oil and beeswax pellets together until the beeswax is completely melted.

4. Remove from heat and let the mixture cool slightly before adding honey and lavender essential oil, if using. Stir well to ensure all ingredients are well combined.

5. Pour the mixture into small tins or jars. Allow it to cool and solidify completely before sealing the containers.

6. Label the containers with the contents and date of preparation.

Variations:

- For a vegan version, substitute beeswax pellets with the same amount of candelilla wax.

- Add vitamin E oil as a natural preservative and to enhance the ointment's skin-healing properties.

- Customize the scent by using different essential oils such as tea tree for additional antimicrobial benefits or chamomile for extra soothing effects.

Storage tips:

Store the calendula ointment in a cool, dry place away from direct sunlight. When stored properly, the ointment can last for up to 1 year. Ensure the containers are tightly sealed to maintain the ointment's efficacy.

Tips for allergens:

Individuals with allergies to plants in the Asteraceae family, including calendula, should perform a patch test before applying the ointment extensively. Substitute olive oil with jojoba or coconut oil if you have sensitivities to olive oil. If allergic to beeswax, using candelilla wax offers a suitable alternative.

120. Arnica Gel

Beneficial effects:

Arnica Gel is widely recognized for its anti-inflammatory and pain-relieving properties, making it an excellent natural remedy for bruises, sprains, muscle aches, and arthritis pain. Its active component, helenalin, is a potent anti-inflammatory agent that helps reduce swelling and pain upon topical application. This makes Arnica Gel an essential component of any herbal first aid kit, providing a safe and effective way to treat minor injuries and relieve pain naturally.

Ingredients:

- 1/4 cup arnica flowers (dried)
- 1/2 cup distilled water
- 1/2 cup aloe vera gel
- 1 tablespoon of witch hazel
- 10 drops of lavender essential oil (optional, for additional pain relief and soothing fragrance)
- 1 teaspoon of vitamin E oil (as a preservative)

Instructions:

1. Begin by infusing the arnica flowers in distilled water. Heat the water to a simmer, add the arnica flowers, and allow to simmer for 30 minutes.

2. After simmering, strain the arnica flowers from the water, squeezing out as much liquid as possible. Discard the flowers.

3. In a mixing bowl, combine the arnica infusion with the aloe vera gel. Stir thoroughly to ensure a homogeneous mixture.

4. Add the witch hazel to the mixture and stir. Witch hazel enhances the gel's anti-inflammatory properties and helps with absorption.

5. If using, add the lavender essential oil and vitamin E oil to the mixture and stir well. These ingredients add soothing properties and act as a preservative.

6. Transfer the Arnica Gel into a clean, sterilized jar. Ensure the jar is dry to avoid contamination.

7. Label the jar with the contents and date of preparation.

Variations:

- For extra cooling relief, add 5 drops of peppermint essential oil to the mixture. Peppermint provides a cooling sensation and further aids in pain relief.

- If a thicker consistency is desired, dissolve 1 teaspoon of natural beeswax in the arnica infusion before mixing it with the aloe vera gel. This will create a more balm-like texture.

Storage tips:

Store the Arnica Gel in the refrigerator to maintain its potency and extend its shelf life. The cool temperature will also provide an additional soothing effect upon application. Use within 6 months for best results.

Tips for allergens:

Individuals with sensitivities to arnica, aloe vera, or any essential oils should perform a patch test on a small area of skin before widespread use. If irritation occurs, discontinue use immediately. For those allergic to lavender, omit the essential oil or substitute with another oil that is well-tolerated, such as chamomile, which also has soothing properties.

121. Lavender Essential Oil

Beneficial effects:

Lavender Essential Oil is celebrated for its calming and soothing properties, making it an invaluable tool in herbal first aid for relieving stress, anxiety, and promoting relaxation. Its antiseptic and anti-inflammatory qualities also make it effective for treating minor burns, cuts, and insect bites, helping to speed up the healing process while reducing pain and preventing infection.

Ingredients:

- 1 cup of carrier oil (such as almond oil, coconut oil, or olive oil)
- 15-20 drops of pure lavender essential oil

Instructions:

1. Choose a clean, dry glass bottle or jar for storage of the lavender essential oil blend.
2. Measure 1 cup of your chosen carrier oil and pour it into the bottle.
3. Add 15-20 drops of pure lavender essential oil to the carrier oil.
4. Secure the lid on the bottle or jar and gently shake to mix the oils thoroughly.
5. Label the bottle with the contents and date of creation.

Variations:

- For enhanced relaxation effects, add 5 drops of chamomile essential oil to the blend.

- To create a more potent antiseptic blend for cuts and scrapes, mix in 5 drops of tea tree oil.

Storage tips:

Store your lavender essential oil blend in a cool, dark place to preserve its potency. When stored properly, the blend can last up to 1 year. Ensure the lid is tightly sealed after each use to prevent oxidation.

Tips for allergens:

Individuals with allergies to nuts should opt for a nut-free carrier oil, such as olive oil. Always perform a patch test on a small area of skin before applying the oil blend extensively, especially if you have sensitive skin or are prone to allergies.

122. Tea Tree Oil Antiseptic

Beneficial effects:

Tea Tree Oil Antiseptic is a natural, powerful remedy for treating cuts, burns, and bites. Its antimicrobial properties help prevent infection, while its anti-inflammatory qualities reduce swelling and pain. This remedy is ideal for quick, effective first aid care, promoting faster healing and reducing the risk of scarring.

Ingredients:

- 2 tablespoons of pure tea tree oil
- 1 cup of distilled water
- A clean spray bottle

Instructions:

1. Pour 1 cup of distilled water into the clean spray bottle.
2. Add 2 tablespoons of pure tea tree oil to the water.

3. Secure the lid on the spray bottle and shake well to mix the ingredients thoroughly.

4. To use, spray the tea tree oil antiseptic directly onto the affected area or apply it with a clean cotton pad.

5. Allow it to air dry. Do not rinse.

6. Apply 2 to 3 times daily until the wound begins to heal.

Variations:

- For sensitive skin, reduce the tea tree oil to 1 tablespoon to make a milder solution.

- Add a tablespoon of aloe vera gel to the mixture for added soothing and healing properties.

- For an extra antimicrobial boost, include a teaspoon of lavender essential oil in the spray.

Storage tips:

Store the tea tree oil antiseptic in a cool, dark place away from direct sunlight. The solution can be kept for up to 1 month. Ensure the spray bottle is tightly closed after each use to maintain the effectiveness of the antiseptic.

Tips for allergens:

Individuals with sensitive skin or allergies to tea tree oil should perform a patch test on a small area of skin before applying the antiseptic widely. If irritation occurs, dilute the mixture with more distilled water or discontinue use.

123. Echinacea Tincture

Beneficial effects:

Echinacea Tincture is widely recognized for its immune-boosting properties, making it an invaluable remedy for preventing and fighting colds, flu, and other respiratory infections. Its active compounds, including alkamides, polysaccharides, and glycoproteins, stimulate the immune system, enhancing the body's ability to combat pathogens. Regular use of Echinacea Tincture can reduce the duration and severity of symptoms, providing natural support for the body's defenses.

Ingredients:

- 1/4 cup dried Echinacea purpurea root
- 1/2 cup 100-proof alcohol (vodka or grain alcohol)

Instructions:

1. Place the dried Echinacea root into a clean, dry jar.

2. Pour the alcohol over the Echinacea, ensuring the roots are completely submerged. Add more alcohol if necessary.

3. Seal the jar tightly and label it with the date and contents.

4. Store the jar in a cool, dark place, shaking it daily, for 4 to 6 weeks. This allows the Echinacea to infuse the alcohol.

5. After the infusion period, strain the tincture through a cheesecloth or fine mesh strainer into another clean, dry jar, pressing the Echinacea to extract as much liquid as possible.

6. Transfer the strained tincture into a dark glass dropper bottle for easy use.

Variations:

- For those sensitive to alcohol, replace vodka with a glycerin and water mixture (3:1 ratio of glycerin to water) to create a non-alcoholic tincture.

- Combine Echinacea with other immune-supporting herbs such as elderberry or astragalus in the tincture for a comprehensive immune-boosting remedy.

Storage tips:

Store the Echinacea Tincture in a cool, dark place. When stored properly, the tincture can last for up to 5 years. Ensure the dropper bottle is tightly sealed to maintain potency.

Tips for allergens:

Individuals with allergies to plants in the daisy family should proceed with caution and may want to consult with a healthcare provider before using Echinacea. Always start with a small dose to ensure no adverse reactions occur.

---

124. Goldenseal Powder

Beneficial effects:

Goldenseal Powder is renowned for its antimicrobial and anti-inflammatory properties, making it an effective natural remedy for a variety of conditions including digestive issues, skin infections, and colds. Its active compound, berberine, has been shown to fight bacteria and viruses, support the immune system, and soothe irritated mucous membranes.

Ingredients:

- 1 teaspoon of goldenseal powder
- 1 cup of boiling water

Instructions:

1. Place 1 teaspoon of goldenseal powder in a cup.
2. Pour 1 cup of boiling water over the goldenseal powder.
3. Stir the mixture well to ensure the powder is fully dissolved.
4. Allow the mixture to steep for 15-20 minutes.
5. Strain the mixture to remove any undissolved particles.
6. Consume the goldenseal tea once it has cooled to a comfortable temperature.

Variations:

- For additional immune support, add a teaspoon of raw honey or lemon juice to the tea after it has steeped.
- Combine goldenseal powder with echinacea tincture in equal parts for a potent immune-boosting remedy.

Storage tips:

Store goldenseal powder in a cool, dry place, away from direct sunlight. Ensure the container is airtight to preserve its potency. Prepared goldenseal tea should be consumed fresh, but can be refrigerated for up to 24 hours if necessary.

Tips for allergens:

Individuals with allergies to plants in the Ranunculaceae family should consult with a healthcare provider before using goldenseal. For those avoiding honey due to allergies or vegan preferences, maple syrup can serve as a sweetening alternative.

125. Witch Hazel Solution

Beneficial effects:

Witch Hazel Solution is a natural remedy renowned for its soothing, anti-inflammatory, and astringent properties. It is particularly effective for treating skin irritations, minor cuts, bruises, and insect bites. By promoting skin healing and reducing inflammation, Witch Hazel Solution can also be used as a gentle toner to cleanse and refresh the skin, making it an essential component of herbal first aid.

Ingredients:

- 1 cup of witch hazel bark
- 2 cups of distilled water
- 1 tablespoon of aloe vera gel (optional, for added soothing effects)

Instructions:

1. Place the witch hazel bark in a small saucepan.

2. Add 2 cups of distilled water to the saucepan and bring to a boil.

3. Reduce the heat and simmer for 30 minutes, allowing the bark to infuse the water.

4. After simmering, remove the saucepan from the heat and allow the mixture to cool to room temperature.

5. Strain the solution through a fine mesh sieve or cheesecloth into a clean bowl, discarding the witch hazel bark.

6. If using, stir in 1 tablespoon of aloe vera gel into the strained witch hazel solution until well combined.

7. Transfer the witch hazel solution into a sterilized glass bottle or jar.

Variations:

- For additional antiseptic properties, add 5 drops of tea tree oil to the solution after it has cooled.

- To enhance the soothing effect, infuse the witch hazel bark with chamomile flowers during the simmering process.

Storage tips:

Store the Witch Hazel Solution in a cool, dark place. If stored properly in a sealed container, it can last for up to 6 months. Ensure the container is tightly sealed to maintain the solution's potency.

Tips for allergens:

For those with sensitivities to aloe vera or tea tree oil, these ingredients can be omitted without significantly affecting the solution's effectiveness. Always perform a patch test on a small area of skin before applying the solution extensively, especially if you have sensitive skin or known allergies.

126. Aloe Vera Burn Gel

Beneficial effects:

Aloe Vera Burn Gel offers immediate cooling relief for burns, cuts, and bites, promoting faster healing and reducing the risk of infection. Aloe vera contains compounds that provide pain relief and decrease inflammation, while its natural gel consistency forms a protective barrier over the wound to keep out bacteria.

Ingredients:

- 1/2 cup of fresh aloe vera gel
- 1 tablespoon of lavender essential oil
- 2 teaspoons of vitamin E oil

Instructions:

1. Extract the gel from an aloe vera leaf by slicing it lengthwise and scooping out the gel with a spoon.

2. Place the fresh aloe vera gel into a blender.

3. Add 1 tablespoon of lavender essential oil to the blender. Lavender oil has natural antiseptic and anti-inflammatory properties, making it an excellent addition for treating skin injuries.

4. Incorporate 2 teaspoons of vitamin E oil, which helps nourish the skin and accelerate the healing process.

5. Blend the mixture on high until it achieves a smooth consistency.

6. Pour the burn gel into a clean, airtight container for storage.

Variations:

- For additional cooling relief, add a few drops of peppermint essential oil to the blend. Peppermint oil provides a cooling sensation that can soothe burns and bites.

- If treating sunburn, mix in a tablespoon of coconut oil for its moisturizing benefits.

Storage tips:

Store the Aloe Vera Burn Gel in the refrigerator for up to one week. The cool temperature will enhance the gel's soothing effect upon application. Ensure the container is sealed tightly to maintain freshness and prevent contamination.

Tips for allergens:

If you have sensitivities to lavender or peppermint essential oil, you can omit these ingredients from the recipe. Aloe vera and vitamin E oil alone still provide significant healing benefits for burns, cuts, and bites. Always perform a patch test on a small area of skin before applying the gel extensively, especially if you have sensitive skin.

127. Calendula Burn Salve

Beneficial effects:

Calendula Burn Salve is known for its remarkable healing properties, particularly suited for treating burns, cuts, and bites. Its anti-inflammatory, antimicrobial, and astringent qualities not only help in reducing pain and swelling but also promote faster healing and prevent infection. The soothing effect of calendula also helps in minimizing scarring, making it an essential remedy for natural wound care.

Ingredients:

- 1/2 cup of dried calendula petals
- 1 cup of coconut oil
- 1/4 cup of beeswax pellets
- 10 drops of lavender essential oil (optional, for added soothing and antimicrobial properties)

Instructions:

1. Combine the dried calendula petals and coconut oil in a double boiler. Heat gently for 2-3 hours to allow the oil to infuse with the calendula's healing properties.
2. Carefully strain the oil through a cheesecloth or fine mesh strainer to remove the calendula petals.
3. Return the infused oil to the double boiler and add the beeswax pellets. Heat until the beeswax is fully melted, stirring continuously.
4. Once the beeswax is melted and mixed with the calendula oil, remove from heat.
5. If using, add the lavender essential oil to the mixture and stir well.
6. Pour the mixture into small tins or jars. Allow it to cool and solidify at room temperature.
7. Once solidified, cover with lids and label the containers with the contents and date.

Variations:

- For a vegan version, replace beeswax with the same amount of candelilla wax.
- Add a few drops of tea tree oil for its powerful antiseptic properties, enhancing the salve's effectiveness in preventing infection.
- Substitute coconut oil with almond oil for a lighter consistency, suitable for sensitive skin.

Storage tips:

Store the Calendula Burn Salve in a cool, dark place. When properly stored, the salve can last for up to 1 year. Ensure the containers are tightly sealed to maintain the salve's therapeutic properties.

Tips for allergens:

Individuals with allergies to plants in the Asteraceae family, including calendula, or those with sensitivities to beeswax, should perform a patch test on a small area of skin before widespread application. Substitute coconut oil with jojoba oil if coconut oil sensitivity is a concern.

128. Plantain Bite Poultice

Beneficial effects:

Plantain Bite Poultice offers natural and effective relief for insect bites, stings, and minor skin irritations. Its anti-inflammatory and antiseptic properties help to soothe the affected area, reduce swelling, and promote healing. Plantain leaves are known for their ability to draw out toxins, making this poultice an excellent choice for treating bites and stings from a variety of insects.

Ingredients:

- A handful of fresh plantain leaves
- Water (as needed to form a paste)
- A clean cloth or gauze

Instructions:

1. Wash the plantain leaves thoroughly to remove any dirt or debris.

2. Crush the leaves using a mortar and pestle or blend them in a food processor with a small amount of water to form a thick paste.

3. Spread the plantain paste directly onto the affected area. If the skin is broken or if you prefer not to apply the paste directly, spread it onto a clean cloth or gauze first.

4. Secure the poultice in place with a bandage or another piece of cloth.

5. Leave the poultice on for up to 2 hours for adults or 1 hour for children. For sensitive skin, check the area frequently and remove sooner if any irritation occurs.

6. After removing, gently wash the area with warm water and pat dry.

Variations:

- For added soothing effects, add a few drops of lavender essential oil to the paste before applying. Lavender oil can help to further reduce inflammation and discomfort.

- If fresh plantain leaves are not available, dried plantain leaves can be rehydrated with warm water and used to create the paste.

Storage tips:

Fresh plantain leaves should be used immediately for the best results. However, if you have leftover leaves, they can be stored in the refrigerator wrapped in a damp paper towel and placed in a plastic bag for up to 2 days. Dried plantain leaves should be stored in an airtight container in a cool, dark place and can last for several months.

Tips for allergens:

If you have known sensitivities to plantain or any added essential oils, it's important to perform a patch test on a small area of skin before applying the poultice widely. In case of an allergic reaction, discontinue use immediately and consult with a healthcare provider if necessary.

129. Yarrow Cut Powder

Beneficial effects:

Yarrow Cut Powder is a natural remedy known for its ability to stop bleeding quickly, making it an invaluable addition to any first aid kit. Its antiseptic and anti-inflammatory properties help to clean wounds, reduce the risk of infection, and support the healing process. Yarrow is also beneficial for treating minor cuts, burns, and insect bites, providing relief and promoting recovery.

Ingredients:

- 1/4 cup dried yarrow flowers and leaves
- Mortar and pestle or a coffee grinder

Instructions:

1. Place the dried yarrow flowers and leaves into a mortar and pestle or a coffee grinder.
2. Grind the yarrow into a fine powder.
3. Store the yarrow cut powder in a small, airtight container.

Variations:

- For additional healing properties, mix the yarrow powder with equal parts of powdered comfrey and plantain. This blend enhances the wound-healing benefits and adds soothing effects for burns and insect bites.

- To create a yarrow paste for direct application to wounds, mix a small amount of the powder with water or honey to form a paste.

Storage tips:

Keep the yarrow cut powder in a cool, dry place, away from direct sunlight. When stored properly in an airtight container, the powder can last for up to a year, retaining its potency and effectiveness.

Tips for allergens:

Individuals with allergies to plants in the Asteraceae family should exercise caution and may want to perform a patch test before using yarrow cut powder on the skin. If an allergic reaction occurs, discontinue use immediately. For those sensitive to pollen, wearing gloves during application may help to avoid potential reactions.

130. Lavender Burn Spray

Beneficial effects:

Lavender Burn Spray provides immediate relief for minor burns, reducing pain, preventing infection, and promoting healing. Lavender essential oil, known for its anti-inflammatory, antiseptic, and soothing properties, helps to calm the skin and accelerate the recovery process. This spray is a must-have for quick and effective first aid treatment for burns, offering a natural alternative to chemical-based products.

Ingredients:

- 1/4 cup distilled water
- 2 tablespoons aloe vera gel
- 10-15 drops lavender essential oil
- 1 teaspoon witch hazel
- Spray bottle for storage

Instructions:

1. In a clean bowl, mix the distilled water and aloe vera gel until well combined. The aloe

vera gel provides a cooling effect and aids in healing the skin.

2. Add 10-15 drops of lavender essential oil to the mixture. Adjust the amount based on the desired strength of the lavender scent and its soothing properties.

3. Incorporate 1 teaspoon of witch hazel into the blend. Witch hazel acts as a natural astringent, helping to cleanse the burn area and reduce inflammation.

4. Pour the mixture into a clean spray bottle. Ensure the bottle is sterilized to prevent contamination.

5. Label the spray bottle with the contents and date of preparation.

Variations:

- For enhanced cooling relief, add 5 drops of peppermint essential oil to the mixture. Peppermint provides a natural cooling sensation, further soothing the burn.

- If the skin is particularly sensitive, reduce the amount of lavender essential oil to prevent any potential irritation.

Storage tips:

Store the Lavender Burn Spray in the refrigerator for an added cooling effect upon application. The cool temperature will also help preserve the active ingredients. Use within 6 months for optimal effectiveness.

Tips for allergens:

Individuals with sensitivities to lavender or witch hazel should perform a patch test on a small area of skin before using the spray extensively. If irritation occurs, dilute the mixture with more distilled water or discontinue use. For those allergic to aloe vera, omit this ingredient and increase the water content to maintain the liquid consistency of the spray.

131. Comfrey Cut Ointment

Beneficial effects:

Comfrey Cut Ointment is a powerful natural remedy for the healing of cuts, burns, and bites. Comfrey, known for its high allantoin content, accelerates cell regeneration, helping wounds to close more quickly and reducing the risk of scarring. Its anti-inflammatory properties also soothe the skin, reducing redness and swelling.

Ingredients:

- 1/4 cup of dried comfrey leaf
- 1/2 cup of coconut oil
- 2 tablespoons of beeswax pellets
- 1 teaspoon of honey (optional, for its antibacterial properties)
- 10 drops of lavender essential oil (optional, for additional antiseptic and soothing effects)

Instructions:

1. In a double boiler, gently melt the coconut oil.

2. Add the dried comfrey leaf to the melted coconut oil and simmer on low heat for 30 minutes to infuse the oil with comfrey's healing properties.

3. Strain the comfrey leaves from the oil using a cheesecloth or fine mesh strainer, squeezing out as much oil as possible. Discard the leaves.

4. Return the infused oil to the double boiler and add the beeswax pellets. Stir until the beeswax is completely melted and well incorporated.

5. Remove from heat and let the mixture cool slightly. If using, stir in the honey and lavender essential oil until fully blended.

6. Pour the mixture into small tins or jars and allow it to solidify at room temperature.

7. Once solidified, seal the containers.

Variations:

- For vegan-friendly ointment, substitute beeswax with an equal amount of candelilla wax.

- Add a few drops of tea tree oil for its powerful antimicrobial properties, especially beneficial for bites and cuts.

Storage tips:

Store the Comfrey Cut Ointment in a cool, dry place. If stored properly, the ointment can last for up to one year. Ensure the containers are tightly sealed to maintain the ointment's effectiveness.

Tips for allergens:

Individuals with sensitivities to comfrey, beeswax, or any essential oils should perform a patch test on a small area of skin before applying the ointment extensively. If irritation occurs, discontinue use. For those allergic to honey, omitting this ingredient will not significantly affect the healing properties of the ointment.

132. Tea Tree Oil Bite Solution

Beneficial effects:

Tea Tree Oil Bite Solution is a natural remedy designed to treat insect bites, providing relief from itching, reducing inflammation, and preventing infection. Tea tree oil, known for its antiseptic, antimicrobial, and anti-inflammatory properties, can quickly soothe the skin, minimize redness, and promote healing.

Ingredients:

- 2 tablespoons of witch hazel
- 10 drops of tea tree essential oil
- 1 tablespoon of aloe vera gel
- 1 teaspoon of honey (optional, for added antimicrobial and soothing properties)

Instructions:

1. In a clean bowl, mix 2 tablespoons of witch hazel with 10 drops of tea tree essential oil.

2. Add 1 tablespoon of aloe vera gel to the mixture and stir until all ingredients are well combined.

3. If using, incorporate 1 teaspoon of honey into the blend for its additional antimicrobial and soothing benefits.

4. Apply a small amount of the solution directly to the insect bite using a cotton ball or a clean fingertip.

5. Allow the solution to dry naturally on the skin. Do not rinse.

6. Apply 2 to 3 times a day until symptoms improve and the bite heals.

Variations:

- For sensitive skin, dilute the tea tree oil by adding an additional tablespoon of witch hazel to the mixture.

- To treat larger areas or multiple bites, double the recipe quantities and store any excess solution in a clean, airtight container for future use.

Storage tips:

Store any leftover Tea Tree Oil Bite Solution in a cool, dark place, ideally in a small glass bottle with a tight-fitting lid. The solution can be kept for up to one week. Ensure the container is properly labeled with the contents and date of preparation.

Tips for allergens:

Individuals with sensitivities to tea tree oil or aloe vera should perform a patch test on a small, unaffected area of skin before applying the solution to bites. If irritation occurs, discontinue use immediately. Honey can be omitted for those with allergies to bee products or for a vegan-friendly version.

133. Goldenseal Cut Powder

Beneficial effects:

Goldenseal Cut Powder is a potent herbal remedy known for its antimicrobial and anti-inflammatory properties, making it highly effective in treating cuts, burns, and bites. By promoting quicker wound healing and reducing the risk of infection, this natural solution supports the body's healing process, ensuring a faster and safer recovery.

Ingredients:

- 2 tablespoons of dried goldenseal root
- 1/2 cup of boiling water

Instructions:

1. Grind the dried goldenseal root into a fine powder using a coffee grinder or mortar and pestle.

2. Place the goldenseal powder in a small bowl.

3. Carefully pour 1/2 cup of boiling water over the goldenseal powder.

4. Stir the mixture until a paste-like consistency is achieved.

5. Allow the paste to cool to a safe temperature for skin application.

6. Apply a thin layer of the goldenseal paste directly to the cleaned cut, burn, or bite.

7. Cover the area with a clean bandage or gauze.

8. Change the dressing and reapply the goldenseal paste once or twice daily until the wound begins to heal.

Variations:

- For enhanced healing properties, mix the goldenseal powder with a teaspoon of honey before adding boiling water. Honey adds additional antimicrobial benefits and can help soothe the skin.

- If treating a burn, you can also blend the goldenseal powder with aloe vera gel instead of water to create a cooling, healing paste.

Storage tips:

Store unused dried goldenseal root in an airtight container in a cool, dark place to maintain its potency. Prepared goldenseal paste should be used immediately, but any leftover paste can be stored in the refrigerator for up to 24 hours in a sealed container.

Tips for allergens:

Individuals with allergies to goldenseal or other herbs should perform a patch test on a small, unaffected area of skin before applying the paste to wounds. If an allergic reaction occurs, discontinue use immediately and consult with a healthcare provider.

134. Witch Hazel Burn Solution

Beneficial effects:

Witch Hazel Burn Solution is a natural remedy known for its soothing and healing properties, particularly effective for treating minor burns, cuts, and insect bites. Its astringent qualities help to reduce inflammation and promote faster healing, while its antimicrobial properties prevent infection. This solution can also provide relief from itching and discomfort associated with skin irritations.

Ingredients:

- 1/2 cup of witch hazel extract
- 1/4 cup of aloe vera gel
- 10 drops of lavender essential oil
- 2 tablespoons of distilled water

Instructions:

1. In a clean bowl, mix the witch hazel extract and distilled water thoroughly.

2. Add the aloe vera gel to the witch hazel mixture and stir until well combined. The aloe vera gel helps soothe the skin and provides a cooling effect on burns.

3. Add 10 drops of lavender essential oil to the mixture. Lavender oil is known for its pain-relieving and anti-inflammatory properties, which can further aid in the healing process of burns and cuts.

4. Pour the solution into a sterilized glass spray bottle or a clean container with a lid.

5. Label the container with the contents and the date of preparation.

Variations:

- For additional cooling relief, you can refrigerate the solution before applying it to the affected area.

- If treating insect bites, you may add 5 drops of tea tree oil for its antiseptic properties.

Storage tips:

Store the Witch Hazel Burn Solution in a cool, dark place or in the refrigerator. When stored properly, the solution can last for up to 6 months. Ensure the container is tightly sealed to maintain the effectiveness of the solution.

Tips for allergens:

Individuals with sensitivities to lavender or other essential oils should perform a patch test on a small area of skin before applying the solution extensively. If irritation occurs, the essential oil can be omitted from the recipe. For those allergic to aloe vera, a simple witch hazel and water solution can also provide relief, though with reduced soothing effects.

135. Echinacea Bite Tincture

Beneficial effects:

Echinacea Bite Tincture is a natural remedy designed to support the body's immune response to insect bites and minor skin irritations. Echinacea, known for its immune-boosting properties, helps reduce inflammation and accelerates the healing process, making it an effective treatment for soothing bites and promoting skin recovery.

Ingredients:

- 1/4 cup dried Echinacea purpurea root
- 1/2 cup 100-proof alcohol (vodka or grain alcohol)

Instructions:

1. Place the dried Echinacea root into a clean, dry jar.

2. Pour the alcohol over the Echinacea, ensuring the roots are completely submerged. Add more alcohol if necessary.

3. Seal the jar tightly and label it with the date and contents.

4. Store the jar in a cool, dark place, shaking it daily, for 4 to 6 weeks. This allows the Echinacea to infuse the alcohol.

5. After the infusion period, strain the tincture through a cheesecloth or fine mesh strainer into another clean, dry jar, pressing the Echinacea to extract as much liquid as possible.

6. Transfer the strained tincture into a dark glass dropper bottle for easy use.

Variations:

- For those sensitive to alcohol, replace vodka with a glycerin and water mixture (3:1 ratio of glycerin to water) to create a non-alcoholic tincture.

- Combine Echinacea with other healing herbs such as calendula or lavender in the tincture for added skin-soothing benefits.

Storage tips:

Store the Echinacea Bite Tincture in a cool, dark place. When stored properly in a sealed container, it can last for up to 5 years. Ensure the dropper bottle is tightly sealed to maintain potency.

Tips for allergens:

Individuals with allergies to plants in the daisy family should consult with a healthcare provider before using Echinacea. Always start with a small dose to ensure no adverse reactions occur.

Part VI: Integrating Herbs into Daily Life

Integrating herbs into daily life offers a transformative approach to health and wellness, empowering individuals to harness nature's healing power in their everyday routines. The journey to incorporating herbal remedies into daily life begins with an understanding of the herbs themselves, recognizing their potential benefits, and learning how to use them safely and effectively. From cooking with herbs to creating simple, homemade remedies, this chapter guides beginners through the process of making herbs a part of their daily lives, enhancing health and well-being naturally.

To start, familiarize yourself with a few key herbs that are known for their versatility and wide range of health benefits. Herbs such as ginger, turmeric, lavender, and peppermint are excellent starting points due to their culinary and medicinal uses. Begin by incorporating these herbs into meals, teas, and as part of your relaxation routines to experience their benefits firsthand.

Objective: To seamlessly integrate herbal practices into daily routines for improved health and wellness.

Preparation:

1. Identify herbs that address specific health needs or interests.

2. Source high-quality, organic herbs from reputable suppliers.

3. Gather basic supplies for preparing herbal remedies and cooking with herbs.

Materials:

- Selected herbs (e.g., ginger, turmeric, lavender, peppermint)

- Carrier oils (for making infused oils)

- Alcohol or vinegar (for tinctures and extracts)

- Beeswax (for salves)

- Glass jars and bottles for storage

Tools:

- Teapot or saucepan

- Strainer or cheesecloth

- Grinder for herbs

- Mixing bowls

- Measuring cups and spoons

Safety measures:

- Always conduct a patch test when trying a new herb topically.

- Consult with a healthcare provider before using herbal remedies, especially if pregnant, nursing, or taking medication.

- Label all homemade remedies with ingredients and date of creation.

Step-by-step Instructions:

1. **Herbal Teas**: Start by making herbal teas. Boil water and pour over a teaspoon of dried herb (or tablespoon if using fresh herbs) per cup. Steep for 5-10 minutes, strain, and enjoy. This can be done daily with herbs like chamomile for relaxation or ginger for digestion.

2. **Cooking with Herbs**: Incorporate herbs into your cooking. Add fresh or dried herbs like rosemary, thyme, or basil to dishes to enhance flavor and nutritional value. Begin with simple recipes that call for herbs you are familiar with.

3. **Herbal Infusions**: Create herbal oils by infusing olive or coconut oil with herbs such as lavender or rosemary. Place herbs in a jar, cover with oil, and let sit in a warm, sunny spot for 2-4 weeks. Strain and use the oil for cooking or as a skin moisturizer.

4. **Making Tinctures**: Fill a jar ⅔ with dried herbs and cover with alcohol or vinegar. Seal and store in a cool, dark place, shaking daily for 4-6 weeks. Strain and store the liquid in a dark bottle. Use a few drops as needed for health benefits.

5. **Crafting Salves**: Melt beeswax and combine with an herbal-infused oil over low heat. Pour into small containers to cool. Label and use for minor skin irritations or as a natural moisturizer.

Cost estimate: Varies, but starting with a few herbs and basic supplies can keep initial costs low.

Time estimate: Preparation times vary; teas can be made in minutes, while tinctures and infusions require several weeks.

Safety tips:

- Keep remedies out of reach of children and pets.

- Be aware of expiration dates for homemade products.

Troubleshooting:

- If an infusion or tincture seems weak, increase the amount of herb or extend the steeping time.

- If a salve is too soft or too hard, adjust the ratio of beeswax to oil and remelt.

Maintenance: Store herbal products in a cool, dark place. Check periodically for signs of spoilage.

Difficulty rating: ★☆☆☆☆ to ★★☆☆☆, depending on the project.

Variations: Experiment with different herbs and combinations to find what works best for your needs and preferences.

By integrating herbs into daily life, individuals can enjoy the myriad benefits that these natural remedies offer. Whether through culinary uses, teas, or homemade remedies, the practice of using herbs daily promotes a holistic approach to health and wellness, empowering individuals to take control of their health in a natural, sustainable way.

Everyday Herbalism

Integrating herbs into daily life is a transformative way to enhance health and wellness, aligning with nature's bounty to support body and mind. Everyday herbalism is about making small, sustainable changes to incorporate the healing power of herbs into the fabric of daily routines. This approach is not only holistic but also accessible, empowering individuals to take proactive steps towards achieving better health naturally.

Objective: To weave herbal practices into the daily lives of individuals, fostering a deeper connection to natural wellness solutions.

Preparation:

- Begin with a reflection on personal and family health goals.
- Identify common ailments or areas for wellness improvement.
- Research herbs that align with these goals.

Materials:

- Kitchen staples (e.g., ginger, garlic, turmeric)
- Essential oils (e.g., lavender, peppermint)
- Fresh or dried herbs (e.g., chamomile, echinacea)
- Carrier oils for infusions (e.g., olive, almond)
- Beeswax for homemade balms and salves

Tools:

- Mason jars for infusions and tinctures
- Tea infuser or French press for herbal teas
- Small pots for creating balms and salves
- Blender or mortar and pestle for herb preparation

Safety measures:

- Verify the identity of all herbs to ensure they are safe for use.
- Understand any potential interactions with medications or health conditions.
- Start with small dosages to monitor reactions.

Step-by-step instructions:

1. **Morning Herbal Tea**: Incorporate a morning ritual of drinking herbal tea. Choose green tea for antioxidants, ginger tea for digestion, or chamomile tea for calming effects. Steep your chosen herb in hot water for 5-10 minutes before enjoying.

2. **Herbal Cooking**: Enhance meals with fresh or dried herbs. Incorporate garlic and turmeric in cooking for their immune-boosting properties. Use basil, oregano, and thyme to add flavor and health benefits to dishes.

3. **Herbal Skincare**: Create a simple lavender oil infusion by soaking lavender buds in a carrier oil for a few weeks. Use this oil as a moisturizer or for stress relief by applying it to the temples or wrists.

4. **Evening Relaxation**: End the day with a calming herbal bath. Add a few drops of chamomile or lavender essential oil to the bathwater, or make a bath tea with oats, lavender, and chamomile for a soothing soak.

Cost estimate: Initial costs may vary, but many herbs can be grown at home or foraged, reducing expenses over time.

Time estimate: Daily practices take minutes to incorporate, while preparing infusions or remedies may require a few weeks for optimal potency.

Safety tips:
- Always dilute essential oils with a carrier oil to prevent skin irritation.
- Keep herbal remedies and essential oils out of reach of children and pets.

Troubleshooting:
- If a skin product causes irritation, discontinue use immediately and consult a healthcare provider.
- If an herb does not provide the desired effect, consider consulting with a herbalist for personalized advice.

Maintenance: Regularly check infusions and remedies for signs of spoilage. Dry herbs should be stored in a cool, dark place to maintain potency.

Difficulty rating: ★☆☆☆☆ for daily practices, ★★☆☆☆ for making simple remedies and infusions.

Variations: Explore different herbs and combinations to find personal favorites and address specific health needs. Experiment with making herbal syrups, vinegars, or honeys for additional ways to incorporate herbs into daily life.

By embracing everyday herbalism, individuals can enjoy a closer connection to the natural world and its healing properties. This practice encourages a holistic view of health, where preventive care and natural remedies work in harmony with the body's own healing abilities. Whether it's starting the day with a refreshing herbal tea, cooking with health-boosting spices, or unwinding with a soothing herbal bath, the integration of herbs into daily routines is a rewarding journey towards enhanced well-being.

Incorporating Herbs into Daily Routine

Incorporating herbs into your daily routine is a simple yet profound way to enhance your health and well-being, connecting with the natural world and tapping into the ancient wisdom of herbal healing. This practice can be seamlessly integrated into your lifestyle, from morning rituals to bedtime routines, offering benefits such as improved digestion, stress reduction, and immune support. Here's how to get started, ensuring that even beginners can confidently and safely make herbs a part of their everyday life.

Objective: To integrate herbal practices into your daily life for health and wellness benefits.

Preparation:

- Identify the health benefits you wish to achieve through herbal remedies.

- Research and select herbs that align with your health goals.

Materials:

- Fresh or dried herbs (e.g., mint, chamomile, lavender, rosemary)

- Essential oils (for aromatherapy)

- Carrier oils (for topical applications)

- Tea infuser or French press

Tools:

- Kettle or pot for boiling water

- Mortar and pestle or blender (for grinding herbs)

- Small jars or bottles (for storing herbal preparations)

Safety measures:

- Always start with small amounts to see how your body reacts.

- Be aware of any potential herb-drug interactions if you are taking medication.

Step-by-step instructions:

1. **Morning**: Begin your day with a herbal tea or tonic. Boil water and steep your chosen herb, such as mint for digestion or green tea for antioxidants, for about 5-10 minutes. This ritual can help set a positive tone for the day ahead.

2. **Cooking**: Incorporate herbs into your meals. Fresh herbs like basil, cilantro, or rosemary can be added to dishes not only to enhance flavor but also to benefit from their health properties. For example, garlic and turmeric have anti-inflammatory qualities.

3. **Work and Study**: Keep a small vial of peppermint essential oil at your desk. A few inhales can help refresh your mind and improve concentration. Alternatively, a lavender oil can reduce stress during hectic moments.

4. **Physical Activity**: Before or after exercise, use a homemade muscle rub made from warming herbs like ginger or cayenne mixed with a carrier oil. Apply to sore areas to help reduce inflammation and soothe muscles.

5. **Evening Relaxation**: Create a bedtime ritual with calming herbs. A cup of chamomile tea or a few drops of lavender essential oil in a diffuser can promote relaxation and better sleep. You can also add Epsom salts and a few drops of essential oils to a warm bath to unwind before bed.

Cost estimate: Initial setup may vary, but many herbs can be grown at home or purchased in bulk to reduce costs.

Time estimate: Daily routines take only a few minutes to incorporate, while preparation times for remedies may vary.

Safety tips:

- Consult a healthcare professional before incorporating new herbs into your routine, especially if you have existing health conditions or are pregnant.

- Always dilute essential oils with a carrier oil before topical application to avoid skin irritation.

Troubleshooting:

- If a tea or remedy seems too strong, dilute it with more water or carrier oil.

- If you experience any adverse reactions, discontinue use immediately and consult a healthcare professional.

Maintenance: Store dried herbs and essential oils in a cool, dark place to preserve their potency. Fresh herbs can be kept in the refrigerator or grown on a windowsill for easy access.

Difficulty rating: ★☆☆☆☆

Variations: Experiment with blending different herbs to create personalized teas and remedies. Each season offers unique herbs to explore and incorporate into your routine, aligning your body with the natural cycles of the year.

By making herbs a part of your daily routine, you embrace a holistic approach to health, grounded in the knowledge that nature provides powerful allies in our journey towards well-being. This practice not only enhances physical health but also nurtures a deeper connection with the environment, encouraging a lifestyle that is both healthful and harmonious with the natural world.

Cooking with Herbs

Cooking with herbs transforms ordinary meals into nourishing, aromatic experiences that can support health and wellness. Herbs, with their diverse flavors and therapeutic properties, offer a simple yet powerful way to enhance both the taste and nutritional value of food. Incorporating herbs into daily cooking routines is an accessible method for harnessing their health benefits, from boosting digestion and immunity to reducing inflammation.

Objective: To integrate health-supportive herbs into everyday meals, making them more flavorful and nutritious.

Preparation:

1. Familiarize yourself with the flavor profiles and health benefits of common culinary herbs such as basil, cilantro, rosemary, thyme, oregano, and parsley.

2. Identify fresh or dried herbs that you can easily incorporate into your current cooking practices.

Materials:

- Fresh or dried culinary herbs

- Olive oil or other carrier oils for infusions

- Garlic, lemon, and other complementary ingredients

Tools:

- Kitchen knife

- Chopping board

- Mortar and pestle or spice grinder (for dried herbs)

- Glass jars for storing herb infusions

Safety measures:

- Ensure fresh herbs are thoroughly washed and dried to remove any pesticides or contaminants.

- When using dried herbs, confirm they are not expired to avoid potential loss of flavor and health benefits.

Step-by-step instructions:

1. **Herb-infused Oils**: Choose a carrier oil (e.g., olive oil) and a combination of herbs. Gently warm the oil without boiling, add herbs, and simmer on low heat for 2-5 minutes. Let the mixture cool, strain, and store in a glass jar. Use for dressings or cooking.

2. **Herbal Seasoning Blends**: Combine dried herbs like rosemary, thyme, and oregano in a mortar and pestle or spice grinder. Grind to a fine consistency. Store in an airtight container and use to season meats, vegetables, or soups.

3. **Fresh Herb Sauces**: Chop fresh herbs such as cilantro, parsley, or basil. Mix with garlic, lemon juice, and olive oil for a vibrant sauce perfect for drizzling over grilled meats or vegetables.

4. **Herb-Infused Water**: Add fresh mint, basil, or cucumber and lemon slices to water. Let it infuse for at least an hour. Enjoy a refreshing and subtly flavored drink.

5. **Baking with Herbs**: Incorporate finely chopped fresh or dried herbs into bread dough, scones, or biscuits for an aromatic twist.

Cost estimate: Minimal, especially if herbs are grown at home or purchased in bulk.

Time estimate: Varies; infusions may take several weeks, while other uses are immediate.

Safety tips:

- Start with small amounts of herbs to ensure the flavor aligns with your preference.

- Always label homemade infusions with the date and ingredients.

Troubleshooting:

- If an infusion tastes too strong, dilute it with more carrier oil.

- If a dish tastes too herbaceous, balance it with a squeeze of lemon juice or a pinch of salt.

Maintenance: Store dried herbs in a cool, dark place. Fresh herbs can last longer if stored in the refrigerator with stems in water.

Difficulty rating: ★☆☆☆☆

Variations: Experiment with different herbs and combinations to discover new flavors and health benefits. For example, try making a sweet basil and mint blend for desserts or a robust rosemary and thyme oil for savory dishes.

Incorporating herbs into your cooking not only elevates the taste of food but also infuses your diet with nature's best medicine. With these simple practices, you can enjoy the therapeutic benefits of herbs in every meal, making each dish a step toward better health and wellness.

Herbal Recipes and Remedies

Creating herbal remedies at home offers a rewarding pathway to natural health and wellness, enabling you to harness the therapeutic powers of plants. This section provides detailed, easy-to-follow recipes and guidelines for crafting your own herbal remedies, from soothing teas to healing salves, each designed to address specific health concerns and enhance overall well-being. Emphasizing safety and simplicity, these recipes are perfect for beginners, using ingredients that are readily accessible and techniques that are straightforward.

136. Herbal Tea for Soothing Sleep

Objective: To promote restful sleep and relaxation.

Preparation:

- Boil 2 cups of water.

- Measure 1 tablespoon of dried chamomile and 1 tablespoon of dried lavender.

Materials:

- Dried chamomile flowers

- Dried lavender flowers

- Water

Tools:

- Kettle or pot

- Teapot or mug

- Strainer

Safety measures: Ensure all herbs are sourced from reputable suppliers to avoid contamination.

Step-by-step instructions:

1. Bring water to a boil in a kettle or pot.

2. Place chamomile and lavender in a teapot or mug.

3. Pour boiling water over the herbs and cover.

4. Steep for 10 minutes.

5. Strain the tea into another cup for drinking.

6. Enjoy a cup 30 minutes before bedtime.

Dosage: One cup before bedtime. Do not exceed two cups per day.

137. Peppermint Digestive Aid

Objective: To relieve digestive discomfort such as bloating and indigestion.

Preparation:

- Boil 1 cup of water.

- Measure 2 teaspoons of dried peppermint leaves.

Materials:

- Dried peppermint leaves

- Water

Tools:

- Kettle or pot

- Teapot or mug

- Strainer

Safety measures: Peppermint may aggravate heartburn in some individuals; start with a small amount to assess tolerance.

Step-by-step instructions:

1. Boil water using a kettle or pot.

2. Add peppermint leaves to a teapot or mug.

3. Pour hot water over the leaves and cover.

4. Steep for 5-7 minutes.

5. Strain and serve.

Dosage: Drink one cup as needed after meals, not exceeding three cups per day.

138. Calendula Salve for Skin Healing

Objective: To facilitate skin healing and soothe irritations.

Preparation:

- Gather all materials and ensure the workspace is clean.

Materials:

- ½ cup of calendula-infused oil
- 2 tablespoons of beeswax pellets
- Vitamin E oil (optional)

Tools:

- Double boiler
- Stirring spoon
- Small jars or tins for storage

Safety measures: Be cautious when handling hot oil and beeswax.

Step-by-step instructions:

1. Heat calendula-infused oil and beeswax in a double boiler over low heat until beeswax melts.

2. Remove from heat and stir in a few drops of vitamin E oil, if using.

3. Pour the mixture into small jars or tins.

4. Allow to cool and solidify before sealing.

5. Label the salve with the date and ingredients.

Dosage: Apply to affected skin areas as needed. Store in a cool, dry place.

139. Ginger Tincture for Nausea

Objective: To alleviate nausea and support digestion.

Preparation:

- Decide on the amount of tincture you wish to make.

- Chop or grate fresh ginger root.

Materials:

- Fresh ginger root
- High-proof alcohol (e.g., vodka)
- Glass jar with a tight-fitting lid

Tools:

- Knife or grater
- Measuring cup
- Strainer or cheesecloth
- Amber dropper bottles for storage

Safety measures: Use food-grade alcohol and ensure proper labeling to avoid misuse.

Step-by-step instructions:

1. Fill a glass jar ⅓ full with chopped or grated ginger.

2. Cover the ginger completely with alcohol, leaving a ½-inch space at the top.

3. Seal the jar tightly and label with the date and contents.

4. Store the jar in a cool, dark place, shaking it daily for 4-6 weeks.

5. After maceration, strain the tincture through a cheesecloth or strainer into a clean bowl.

6. Transfer the strained tincture into amber dropper bottles.

7. Label the bottles with the date and contents.

Dosage: Take 1-2 ml, up to three times daily, diluted in water or juice.

These herbal recipes and remedies offer a foundation for exploring the vast world of herbal medicine. With practice and patience, you can expand your repertoire, tailoring remedies to meet your unique health needs and preferences. Remember to consult with a healthcare provider before adding new herbal remedies to your routine, especially if you have existing health conditions or are taking medications.

140. Elderberry and Ginger Tonic

Beneficial effects:

Elderberry and Ginger Tonic is a potent blend designed to boost the immune system, alleviate cold and flu symptoms, and promote overall wellness. Elderberries are rich in vitamins and antioxidants, which can help fight inflammation and protect against viruses and bacteria. Ginger adds digestive and anti-inflammatory benefits, making this tonic an excellent choice for enhancing immune response and soothing respiratory conditions.

Ingredients:

- 1/2 cup dried elderberries
- 2 tablespoons freshly grated ginger
- 4 cups of water
- 1 cup raw honey
- Juice of 1 lemon

Instructions:

1. Combine the dried elderberries, grated ginger, and water in a medium saucepan.

2. Bring the mixture to a boil, then reduce heat and simmer for about 20 minutes, allowing the ingredients to infuse their properties into the water.

3. Remove from heat and let the mixture cool to room temperature.

4. Strain the mixture through a fine mesh sieve or cheesecloth into a large bowl, pressing on the solids to extract as much liquid as possible.

5. Stir in the raw honey and lemon juice until well combined.

6. Transfer the tonic to a clean glass bottle or jar and seal tightly.

Variations:

- For an extra immune boost, add a teaspoon of ground turmeric to the mixture during the simmering process.
- Replace raw honey with maple syrup for a vegan-friendly version.
- Add a cinnamon stick during the simmering process for additional flavor and health benefits.

Storage tips:

Store the Elderberry and Ginger Tonic in the refrigerator for up to two weeks. Shake well before each use as natural separation may occur.

Tips for allergens:

Individuals with allergies to pollen or bee products should substitute honey with maple syrup to avoid allergic reactions. Always ensure that the elderberries and ginger are sourced from reputable suppliers to avoid contamination with allergens.

141. Lemon and Turmeric Elixir

Beneficial effects:

The Lemon and Turmeric Elixir is a potent detoxifying and immune-boosting drink. Turmeric, with its active ingredient curcumin, offers powerful anti-inflammatory and antioxidant benefits, while lemon is rich in vitamin C, aiding in detoxification and enhancing the immune system. This elixir supports liver function, aids in digestion, and can help in reducing inflammation throughout the body.

Ingredients:

- 1 tablespoon of turmeric powder
- Juice of 1 lemon
- 1 tablespoon of raw honey
- A pinch of black pepper (to enhance curcumin absorption)
- 2 cups of warm water

Instructions:

1. Warm 2 cups of water to a comfortable drinking temperature.
2. Add 1 tablespoon of turmeric powder and a pinch of black pepper to the warm water.
3. Squeeze the juice of 1 lemon into the mixture.
4. Stir in 1 tablespoon of raw honey until fully dissolved.
5. Consume the elixir warm, preferably on an empty stomach in the morning to maximize its detoxifying benefits.

Variations: - For an added boost, include a teaspoon of grated ginger to the drink for its digestive and anti-inflammatory benefits.

- Replace warm water with green tea for an extra antioxidant kick.
- For those who prefer a cold beverage, allow the drink to cool and serve over ice.

Storage tips:

This detox drink is best consumed fresh to ensure the potency of its ingredients. However, if preparing in advance, store it in the refrigerator in a glass container for up to 24 hours. Shake well before consuming.

Tips for allergens:

Individuals with allergies to pollen or bee products should substitute honey with maple syrup or simply omit the sweetener. Those with a sensitivity to turmeric or black pepper should adjust the quantities according to their tolerance or consult with a healthcare provider before incorporating this drink into their routine.

142. Rosemary and Lemon Balm Tonic

Beneficial effects:

Rosemary and Lemon Balm Tonic is a refreshing and therapeutic drink that combines the cognitive-boosting properties of rosemary with the calming effects of lemon balm. This tonic is ideal for enhancing memory, focus, and mental clarity while also providing a soothing effect on the nervous system, making it perfect for stress relief and relaxation. Additionally, both herbs have antioxidant properties that support overall health and well-being.

Ingredients:

- 1 tablespoon of fresh rosemary leaves
- 1 tablespoon of fresh lemon balm leaves
- 2 cups of boiling water
- Honey or lemon to taste (optional)

Instructions:

1. Place the fresh rosemary and lemon balm leaves in a heat-resistant pitcher or teapot.
2. Pour 2 cups of boiling water over the herbs.
3. Cover and allow the mixture to steep for 10 to 15 minutes.
4. Strain the tonic to remove the leaves.
5. If desired, add honey or lemon to taste.
6. Serve the tonic warm, or allow it to cool and enjoy it chilled.

Variations:

- For a cold beverage option, allow the tea to cool to room temperature, then refrigerate for 1-2 hours. Serve over ice if desired.
- Add slices of fresh ginger during the steeping process for an additional detoxifying effect and a spicy kick.
- Combine with green tea for an extra boost of antioxidants.

Storage tips:

The Rosemary and Lemon Balm Tonic can be stored in the refrigerator for up to 48 hours. Keep it in a sealed glass container to maintain freshness and prevent absorption of other flavors from the fridge.

Tips for allergens:

For those with specific plant allergies, ensure that both rosemary and lemon balm are suitable for your consumption. For those avoiding honey due to allergies or vegan preferences, stevia or agave syrup can serve as alternative sweeteners.

143. Ginger and Mint Elixir

Beneficial effects:

The Ginger and Mint Elixir is designed to soothe the digestive system, reduce inflammation, and boost immunity. Ginger, with its powerful anti-inflammatory properties, helps alleviate nausea, indigestion, and menstrual discomfort. Mint contributes a refreshing flavor while promoting digestion and relieving symptoms of irritable bowel syndrome (IBS). Together, they create a potent tonic that not only supports digestive health but also strengthens the body's defense mechanisms.

Ingredients:

- 1 tablespoon of freshly grated ginger
- 1 tablespoon of fresh mint leaves, finely chopped
- 2 cups of boiling water
- 1 tablespoon of honey (optional, for sweetness)
- Juice of half a lemon

Instructions:

1. Place the freshly grated ginger and chopped mint leaves in a heat-resistant pitcher or teapot.
2. Pour 2 cups of boiling water over the ginger and mint.
3. Cover and allow the mixture to steep for 10 to 15 minutes.
4. Strain the elixir into cups, removing the ginger and mint leaves.
5. Stir in the honey (if using) until dissolved, and add the lemon juice for an extra vitamin C boost.
6. Serve the elixir warm, or allow it to cool and serve over ice for a refreshing drink.

Variations:

- For an added immune boost, include a pinch of turmeric powder to the elixir while it steeps.
- Replace honey with maple syrup for a vegan-friendly sweetener option.
- Add a slice of cucumber or a few slices of apple for a subtle flavor twist and added health benefits.

Storage tips:

This elixir is best enjoyed fresh to maximize the benefits of the ingredients. However, if you need to store it, keep it in a sealed glass container in the refrigerator for up to 24 hours. Gently reheat without boiling or enjoy chilled.

Tips for allergens:

Individuals with allergies to ginger or mint should adjust the recipe accordingly or consult with a healthcare provider before consuming. For those with sensitivities to honey, maple syrup serves as a suitable alternative that maintains the elixir's beneficial properties.

144. Holy Basil and Lemon Tonic

Beneficial effects:

Holy Basil and Lemon Tonic is a revitalizing drink that harnesses the stress-reducing and immune-boosting properties of Holy Basil, combined with the detoxifying and vitamin C-rich benefits of lemon. This tonic is designed to support overall well-being, enhance mental clarity, and promote a balanced mood, making it an excellent daily elixir for maintaining health and vitality.

Ingredients:

- 1 tablespoon of dried Holy Basil leaves
- Juice of 1 lemon
- 1 teaspoon of raw honey (optional)
- 2 cups of boiling water

Instructions:

1. Place the dried Holy Basil leaves in a heat-resistant pitcher or teapot.

2. Add the juice of 1 lemon to the pitcher.

3. Pour 2 cups of boiling water over the Holy Basil leaves and lemon juice.

4. Allow the mixture to steep for 5-10 minutes.

5. Strain the tonic into cups, discarding the Holy Basil leaves.

6. Stir in 1 teaspoon of raw honey, if desired, until fully dissolved.

7. Serve the tonic warm, or allow it to cool and enjoy it as a refreshing cold beverage.

Variations:

- For a caffeine boost, mix the tonic with green tea, allowing both to steep together before straining.

- Add a slice of fresh ginger during the steeping process for an additional anti-inflammatory boost and a spicy flavor.

- Substitute honey with maple syrup for a vegan-friendly sweetener option.

Storage tips:

The Holy Basil and Lemon Tonic is best enjoyed fresh. However, if you need to store it, keep it in a refrigerator in a sealed glass container for up to 24 hours. Reheat gently on the stove or enjoy cold.

Tips for allergens:

Individuals with sensitivities to herbs should start with a smaller amount of Holy Basil to ensure tolerance. For those avoiding honey due to allergies or dietary preferences, maple syrup serves as a suitable alternative without compromising the tonic's beneficial properties.

145. Sage and Lavender Elixir

Beneficial effects:

Sage and Lavender Elixir harnesses the calming and soothing properties of both sage and lavender, making it an excellent remedy for reducing stress, anxiety, and promoting relaxation. Sage is known for its antioxidant and anti-inflammatory benefits, while lavender adds to the calming effect, aiding in better sleep and mood enhancement.

Ingredients:

- 2 tablespoons of fresh sage leaves
- 1 tablespoon of dried lavender flowers
- 2 cups of boiling water
- Honey or lemon to taste (optional)

Instructions:

1. Place the fresh sage leaves and dried lavender flowers in a large teapot or heat-resistant pitcher.

2. Pour 2 cups of boiling water over the sage and lavender.

3. Cover and allow the mixture to steep for 5 to 10 minutes, depending on the desired strength.

4. Strain the elixir into cups, discarding the sage leaves and lavender flowers.

5. If desired, add honey or lemon to taste for additional flavor.

6. Serve the elixir warm, or allow it to cool and enjoy it chilled.

Variations:

- For a refreshing summer drink, let the elixir cool to room temperature, then refrigerate for 1-2 hours and serve over ice.

- Add a slice of fresh ginger during the steeping process for an additional digestive benefit and a spicy kick.

- Mix in a teaspoon of apple cider vinegar to the cooled elixir for a detoxifying boost.

Storage tips:

The Sage and Lavender Elixir is best enjoyed fresh. However, if you need to store it, keep it in a sealed glass container in the refrigerator for up to 24 hours. Reheat gently on the stove or enjoy cold.

Tips for allergens:

Individuals with sensitivities to sage or lavender should start with a smaller amount to ensure no adverse reactions occur. For those avoiding honey due to allergies or vegan preferences, maple syrup can serve as a sweetening alternative.

146. Peppermint and Lemon Tonic

Beneficial effects:

Peppermint and Lemon Tonic serves as a refreshing and revitalizing drink that aids in digestion, boosts the immune system, and provides a natural energy lift. Peppermint is known for its ability to soothe the stomach and improve digestive health, while lemon is rich in Vitamin C, detoxifying the body and enhancing immune function. This tonic is perfect for daily consumption to maintain overall well-being and vitality.

Ingredients:

- 1/4 cup of fresh peppermint leaves
- Juice of 1 lemon
- 1 tablespoon of honey (optional, for sweetness)
- 2 cups of boiling water
- Ice cubes (for serving)

Instructions:

1. Place the fresh peppermint leaves in a large mug or heatproof container.

2. Add the juice of 1 lemon to the mug.

3. If using, stir in 1 tablespoon of honey for added sweetness.

4. Pour 2 cups of boiling water over the peppermint leaves and lemon juice.

5. Allow the mixture to steep for 5-10 minutes, depending on the desired strength.

6. Strain the tonic to remove the peppermint leaves.

7. Serve the tonic warm or allow it to cool and serve over ice cubes for a refreshing drink.

Variations:

- For an extra immune boost, add a slice of fresh ginger to the tonic while it steeps.
- Substitute honey with maple syrup for a vegan-friendly version.
- Add a dash of cayenne pepper for a drink with a kick that can further boost metabolism.

Storage tips:

The Peppermint and Lemon Tonic can be stored in the refrigerator for up to 24 hours. Keep it in a sealed glass container to maintain freshness and prevent absorption of other flavors from the fridge.

Tips for allergens:

Individuals with allergies to peppermint or citrus should adjust the recipe according to their dietary needs or consult with a healthcare provider before consuming. For those avoiding honey due to allergies or dietary preferences, maple syrup serves as a suitable alternative without compromising the tonic's health benefits.

147. Chamomile and Ginger Elixir

Beneficial effects:

The Chamomile and Ginger Elixir combines the soothing properties of chamomile with the digestive and anti-inflammatory benefits of ginger, creating a powerful tonic that can help reduce stress, alleviate digestive issues, and boost the immune system. Chamomile is known for its calming effects, which can aid in improving sleep quality and reducing anxiety. Ginger, on the other hand, is a potent anti-inflammatory agent that can help relieve nausea, fight colds, and soothe sore throats.

Ingredients:

- 2 tablespoons of dried chamomile flowers
- 1 inch of fresh ginger root, thinly sliced
- 4 cups of boiling water
- Honey or lemon to taste (optional)

Instructions:

1. Place the dried chamomile flowers and thinly sliced ginger in a large teapot or heatproof pitcher.

2. Pour 4 cups of boiling water over the chamomile and ginger.

3. Cover and allow the mixture to steep for 10 minutes.

4. Strain the elixir into mugs or glasses, discarding the chamomile and ginger.

5. If desired, add honey or lemon to taste for additional flavor.

6. Serve the elixir warm or allow it to cool and serve over ice for a refreshing drink.

Variations:

- For an added immune boost, include a teaspoon of turmeric powder to the elixir while it steeps.

- To enhance the calming effects, add a few sprigs of fresh mint to the mixture before steeping.

- For a sweeter version without added sugars, blend in a small apple or pear before straining.

Storage tips:

The Chamomile and Ginger Elixir is best enjoyed fresh. However, it can be stored in the refrigerator in a sealed container for up to 24 hours. Reheat gently on the stove or enjoy chilled.

Tips for allergens:

Individuals with allergies to chamomile (which is part of the daisy family) or ginger should exercise caution and may want to consult with a healthcare provider before consuming this elixir. Honey can be substituted with maple syrup for those with allergies to bee products or for a vegan-friendly option.

148. Thyme and Lemon Tonic

Beneficial effects:

Thyme and Lemon Tonic serves as a refreshing and therapeutic drink, aimed at boosting the immune system, alleviating symptoms of colds and coughs, and promoting digestive health. Thyme is known for its antibacterial and antiviral properties, making it effective in fighting respiratory infections. Lemon, rich in vitamin C, aids in detoxification and strengthens the immune system, while also providing a zesty flavor that invigorates the senses.

Ingredients:

- 2 tablespoons of fresh thyme leaves
- Juice of 1 lemon
- 1 tablespoon of raw honey (optional, for sweetness)
- 2 cups of boiling water

Instructions:

1. Place the fresh thyme leaves in a teapot or heatproof pitcher.
2. Add the juice of 1 lemon to the thyme.
3. Pour 2 cups of boiling water over the thyme and lemon juice.
4. Cover and allow the mixture to steep for 10 to 15 minutes.
5. Strain the tonic into cups or a serving pitcher.
6. Stir in 1 tablespoon of raw honey, if using, until dissolved.
7. Serve the tonic warm, or allow it to cool and serve over ice for a refreshing drink.

Variations:

- For an added immune boost, include a slice of fresh ginger or a pinch of cayenne pepper while steeping.
- Replace honey with maple syrup for a vegan-friendly version.
- Add a sprig of mint for a refreshing twist.

Storage tips:

This tonic is best enjoyed fresh. However, if you need to store it, keep it in a sealed glass container in the refrigerator for up to 24 hours. Reheat gently on the stove or enjoy chilled.

Tips for allergens:

Individuals with allergies to citrus can omit the lemon juice and substitute it with apple cider vinegar for a similar detoxifying effect. For those with sensitivities to honey, maple syrup serves as a suitable alternative that maintains the tonic's beneficial properties.

149. Dandelion and Ginger Elixir

Beneficial effects:

The Dandelion and Ginger Elixir harnesses the detoxifying power of dandelion and the anti-inflammatory benefits of ginger, creating a potent tonic that supports liver health, aids digestion, and boosts the immune system. Dandelion is known for its ability to cleanse the liver and eliminate toxins, while ginger reduces inflammation and soothes the digestive tract, making this elixir an excellent choice for promoting overall wellness.

Ingredients:

- 1 tablespoon of dried dandelion root
- 1 inch piece of fresh ginger, thinly sliced
- 2 cups of boiling water
- 1 teaspoon of raw honey (optional, for sweetness)
- Juice of 1/2 lemon (optional, for added detoxifying benefits and flavor)

Instructions:

1. Place the dried dandelion root and sliced ginger in a heat-resistant container or teapot.
2. Pour 2 cups of boiling water over the dandelion and ginger.
3. Cover and allow the mixture to steep for 10 to 15 minutes.
4. Strain the elixir into a mug or glass, removing the dandelion root and ginger pieces.
5. If desired, stir in the raw honey and lemon juice until well combined.
6. Enjoy the elixir warm, or allow it to cool and drink it as a refreshing cold beverage.

Variations:

- For an extra immune boost, add a pinch of ground turmeric to the elixir during the steeping process. Turmeric's curcumin content offers additional anti-inflammatory and antioxidant benefits.
- Replace raw honey with maple syrup for a vegan-friendly sweetener option.
- Add a cinnamon stick to the boiling water for a warming spice flavor that also has blood sugar-regulating properties.

Storage tips:

This elixir is best enjoyed fresh to maximize the benefits of its ingredients. However, if you need to store it, keep it in a sealed glass container in the refrigerator for up to 24 hours. Reheat gently on the stove or enjoy chilled.

Tips for allergens:

Those with allergies to ragweed or other related plants should be cautious when consuming dandelion and may want to consult with a healthcare provider before trying this elixir. For individuals sensitive to honey, maple syrup serves as a suitable alternative that maintains the elixir's beneficial properties.

Healing Beverages

Healing beverages harness the power of herbs to support overall health, offering a delightful and therapeutic way to hydrate and nourish the body. These drinks, ranging from teas and infusions to tonics and elixirs, incorporate a variety of medicinal plants known for their healing properties. Each recipe provided here is designed to be both accessible to beginners and beneficial for a wide range of health concerns, from boosting the immune system to calming the nerves.

Objective: To create simple, healing beverages that utilize the natural benefits of herbs to enhance well-being.

Preparation:

- Select the herbs based on the desired health benefit.

- Clean and prepare the workspace and utensils.

Materials:

- Fresh or dried herbs (e.g., mint, chamomile, ginger, turmeric)

- Natural sweeteners (optional, such as honey or stevia)

- Additional ingredients for flavor and health benefits (e.g., lemon, cinnamon, elderberry)

Tools:

- Teapot or saucepan

- Strainer or tea infuser

- Measuring cups and spoons

- Kettle for boiling water

Safety measures:

- Verify the safety of herbs for individual health conditions and potential interactions with medications.

- Ensure all herbs are correctly identified and sourced from reputable suppliers.

Step-by-step Instructions:

1. **Mint and Lemon Digestive Aid**:

- Boil 2 cups of water.

- Add 1 tablespoon of fresh or dried mint leaves and a few slices of lemon.

- Steep for 5-10 minutes, then strain.

- Sweeten with honey if desired.

2. **Chamomile Sleep Tonic**:

- Boil 2 cups of water.

- Add 2 tablespoons of dried chamomile flowers.

- Cover and steep for 10 minutes, then strain.
- Drink 30 minutes before bedtime for a restful sleep.

3. **Ginger-Turmeric Immune Booster**:
- Boil 2 cups of water with 1 inch of ginger root, sliced, and 1 teaspoon of turmeric powder.
- Simmer for 10 minutes.
- Strain and add honey and a squeeze of lemon juice to taste.

4. **Elderberry Cold and Flu Elixir**:
- Simmer 2 tablespoons of dried elderberries in 3 cups of water for 30 minutes.
- Strain and add 1 tablespoon of honey or to taste.
- Drink warm to boost immunity and soothe cold symptoms.

Cost estimate: Minimal, especially if herbs are grown at home or foraged.

Time estimate: Most beverages can be prepared in 15-30 minutes, including brewing time.

Safety tips:
- Always start with a small amount to test for any adverse reactions.
- Consult a healthcare professional before regularly incorporating new herbal beverages into your diet, especially for children, pregnant or nursing women, and those with medical conditions.

Troubleshooting:
- If a beverage is too strong, dilute it with more water.
- If not flavorful enough, increase the amount of herbs or steeping time on the next preparation.

Maintenance: Dried herbs should be stored in a cool, dark place in airtight containers to preserve their potency.

Difficulty rating: ★☆☆☆☆

Variations: Feel free to experiment with combining different herbs to tailor the flavor and health benefits to personal preferences. For example, adding lavender to the Chamomile Sleep Tonic can enhance its relaxing effects, while mixing cinnamon with the Ginger-Turmeric Immune Booster can provide additional antioxidant benefits.

By incorporating these healing beverages into daily routines, individuals can enjoy the therapeutic qualities of herbs in a delicious and comforting form. These recipes are just the beginning, inviting exploration into the vast world of herbal remedies and the many ways they can support health and wellness.

DIY Beauty Products

Creating your own DIY beauty products is a rewarding and empowering way to use the healing power of herbs for skin and hair care. With simple, natural ingredients and a few basic tools, you can craft a range of products from moisturizers and toners to shampoos and conditioners that are tailored to your specific beauty needs. These homemade creations not only reduce exposure to harmful chemicals found in many commercial products but also offer a sustainable, cost-effective approach to beauty.

Objective: To craft natural, effective beauty products using herbal ingredients.

Preparation:

- Decide on the type of beauty product you wish to create.

- Research herbs and natural ingredients beneficial for your skin or hair type.

Materials:

- Herbs (e.g., chamomile for soothing, rosemary for hair growth)

- Carrier oils (e.g., coconut oil, jojoba oil)

- Essential oils for fragrance and added benefits (e.g., lavender for relaxation, tea tree for acne)

- Beeswax or shea butter for balms and creams

- Distilled water or herbal teas as bases for toners and shampoos

- Aloe vera gel for soothing and moisturizing products

Tools:

- Double boiler for melting waxes and oils

- Blender or food processor for mixing

- Sieve or cheesecloth for straining herbal infusions

- Measuring cups and spoons

- Jars, bottles, and containers for storage

Safety measures:

- Conduct a patch test with the finished product to check for any allergic reactions.

- Ensure all containers and tools are sterilized to prevent contamination.

Step-by-step instructions:

1. **Herbal Infused Oil**:

- Gently heat 1 cup of carrier oil with ¼ cup of dried herbs of your choice in a double boiler for 2-3 hours on low heat.

- Strain the mixture through a cheesecloth into a clean jar. This infused oil can be used as a base for various beauty products.

2. Moisturizing Herbal Cream:

- Melt 2 tablespoons of beeswax into ½ cup of herbal infused oil.
- Slowly add ¼ cup of distilled water or herbal tea, stirring constantly until well blended.
- Allow to cool slightly before adding 10-15 drops of essential oil.
- Pour into a clean jar and let it set.

3. Natural Herbal Shampoo:

- Brew a strong herbal tea with herbs that match your hair type (e.g., nettle for hair growth, chamomile for highlights).
- Mix ½ cup of herbal tea with ½ cup of castile soap and 1 teaspoon of carrier oil.
- Add up to 20 drops of essential oil for fragrance and additional benefits.
- Store in a bottle and shake well before each use.

4. Soothing Herbal Toner:

- Brew a cup of herbal tea using herbs like rose, chamomile, or green tea.
- Allow the tea to cool, then mix with equal parts witch hazel.
- Add a few drops of essential oil if desired.
- Store in a clean bottle and use with a cotton pad after cleansing.

Cost estimate: Varies, but generally low to moderate, depending on the choice of herbs and oils.

Time estimate: Preparation time ranges from 30 minutes to 3 hours, depending on the product.

Safety tips:

- Label all products with ingredients and the date of creation.
- Store products in a cool, dark place to preserve their potency.

Troubleshooting:

- If a cream or balm is too thick, reheat and add more oil or distilled water.
- If a shampoo or toner is too mild, increase the concentration of herbs or essential oils.

Maintenance: Check products regularly for any changes in smell, texture, or color, which could indicate spoilage.

Difficulty rating: ★☆☆☆☆ to ★★☆☆☆, depending on the complexity of the product.

Variations: Experiment with different combinations of herbs and oils to create customized products that cater to your specific beauty concerns. For example, switch rosemary for peppermint in the shampoo recipe for a refreshing scalp treatment or use shea butter instead of beeswax for a creamier texture in balms and creams.

By taking the time to create your own DIY beauty products, you not only gain control over the ingredients that come into contact with your body but also have the opportunity to connect with the healing power of nature. These homemade beauty solutions offer a mindful, personalized approach to skincare and haircare that can be both fulfilling and fun.

Conclusion

Embracing the journey through the world of herbal remedies opens up a new horizon for enhancing health and well-being naturally. This exploration into the healing power of plants has equipped you with the knowledge to incorporate herbal remedies into your everyday life, providing a foundation for a healthier, more holistic approach to living. As you continue to experiment with and integrate these natural solutions, remember the importance of sourcing high-quality ingredients, understanding proper dosages, and respecting the wisdom of nature.

The path to natural healing is both personal and universal, connecting us to the ancient traditions of herbal medicine while inviting us to innovate and personalize our approach to wellness. Whether it's crafting a soothing chamomile tea to unwind before bed, applying a lavender salve to calm the skin, or sipping on ginger lemon tea to bolster the immune system, the power of plants is profound and multifaceted.

As you move forward, let curiosity be your guide. Experiment with different herbs and remedies to discover what works best for you and your family. Share your successes and learnings with the community, contributing to a collective knowledge base that enriches our understanding and application of herbal medicine.

The journey doesn't end here; it evolves with each new discovery and insight into the natural world. Continue to seek out information, attend workshops, and connect with herbalists and fellow enthusiasts to deepen your practice. The Lost Bible of Herbal Remedies is not just a guide but a companion on your path to natural health, offering a gateway to a life enriched by the wisdom of herbs.

In this quest for well-being, remember that the most profound healing comes from aligning with nature, listening to our bodies, and nurturing our connection to the earth. Here's to your health, happiness, and the endless exploration of the healing power of plants.

Living Naturally

Living naturally embodies a lifestyle that harmonizes with the earth's rhythms and cycles, prioritizing wellness through the purity of nature's bounty. Embracing this way of life means making conscious choices that enhance health and well-being, not just for the individual but for the planet as a whole. It involves integrating herbal remedies into daily routines, choosing organic and locally sourced foods, reducing reliance on synthetic products, and fostering a deep connection with the environment. This holistic approach to living encourages a mindful interaction with the world, promoting a life of balance, health, and sustainability.

To embark on this journey towards living naturally, begin by incorporating more plant-based foods into your diet, rich in nutrients and naturally detoxifying properties. Cultivate a garden, no matter the size, to connect with the cycle of growth and harvest, understanding firsthand the source of your food and remedies. When gardening, choose non-GMO seeds and organic practices that support soil health and biodiversity.

Engage in regular physical activities that connect you with nature, such as hiking, yoga, or simply walking barefoot on the earth, to ground yourself and enhance physical fitness. These activities not only improve physical health but also mental well-being, reducing stress and fostering a sense of peace.

Incorporate herbal remedies into your healthcare regimen to address common ailments, relying on the healing power of plants to nurture your body back to health. Start with simple recipes, such as herbal teas and tinctures, to naturally support your body's immune system, digestive health, and stress response. Always prioritize safety by understanding the proper use of each herb, including potential interactions with medications and individual health conditions.

Reduce your environmental footprint by choosing eco-friendly and sustainable products, from household cleaners to personal care items. Opt for products packaged in biodegradable or recyclable materials and consider making your own natural alternatives using simple ingredients like vinegar, baking soda, and essential oils.

Living naturally also means being part of a community that shares your values and supports your journey. Engage with local herbalists, join gardening clubs, or participate in community-supported agriculture (CSA) programs to deepen your connection with like-minded individuals and the local ecosystem.

By adopting a lifestyle that values simplicity, health, and sustainability, you not only enhance your own well-being but also contribute to the health of the planet. Living naturally is an empowering choice that aligns your actions with your values, leading to a fulfilling and harmonious life.

The Future of Herbal Medicine

The future of herbal medicine holds immense potential as it continues to blend ancient wisdom with modern scientific understanding, offering a promising avenue for holistic health care. As we move forward, the integration of herbal remedies into mainstream healthcare systems is becoming more prevalent, driven by a growing body of research that validates the efficacy and safety of plant-based treatments. This evolution is not just about revisiting traditional practices but about advancing them through rigorous scientific methodologies to ensure they meet contemporary health needs effectively and safely.

Technological advancements are set to play a pivotal role in the future of herbal medicine. Innovations in extraction and preservation techniques will enhance the potency and shelf life of herbal remedies, making them more accessible and convenient for everyday use. Furthermore, the development of sophisticated analytical tools will allow for a deeper understanding of the complex chemical compositions of medicinal plants, unlocking new therapeutic potentials and enabling the customization of remedies to suit individual health profiles.

Sustainability will be at the heart of the future of herbal medicine. As demand for herbal remedies grows, there will be an increased focus on ethical sourcing, cultivation, and harvesting practices to protect biodiversity and ensure the long-term availability of medicinal plants. This will involve a collaborative effort among herbalists, conservationists, and local communities to promote regenerative agriculture practices that replenish and nurture the earth.

Education and awareness will also be key components of the future of herbal medicine. There will be a greater emphasis on educating healthcare professionals about the benefits and uses of herbal remedies, fostering a more integrated approach to health care. At the same time, public education initiatives will empower individuals with the knowledge to make informed decisions about their health, encouraging a proactive approach to wellness that emphasizes prevention and self-care.

In the realm of regulation, we can anticipate more standardized guidelines for the production, labeling, and distribution of herbal products. This will enhance consumer trust and safety, ensuring that herbal remedies are held to the same high standards as conventional medicines. Such regulations will also support the credibility and growth of the herbal medicine industry, paving the way for more widespread acceptance and use of plant-based treatments.

As we look to the future, the role of community and collaboration becomes ever more critical. The collective wisdom of traditional healers, modern herbalists, scientists, and educators will drive the evolution of herbal medicine, creating a more inclusive and holistic health care system. This collaborative spirit, coupled with a shared commitment to sustainability and wellness, will ensure that the ancient art of herbal healing continues to thrive, offering hope and healing for generations to come.

In embracing the future of herbal medicine, we are not merely turning back to the past; we are moving forward with a renewed appreciation for the healing power of nature, grounded in science and guided by a vision of health and harmony for all.

Resources and References

For those eager to delve deeper into the world of herbal remedies and natural healing, a wealth of resources and references awaits. The journey into herbalism is enriched by exploring a variety of sources, from classic texts that lay the groundwork of herbal knowledge to modern studies that offer the latest insights into plant-based healing.

Key references include seminal works such as "The Complete Herbal" by Nicholas Culpeper, which provides a historical perspective on the uses of herbs, and "Medical Herbalism" by David Hoffmann, which bridges the gap between traditional herbalism and contemporary science. For those interested in the scientific underpinnings of herbal medicine, "Principles and Practice of Phytotherapy" by Kerry Bone and Simon Mills offers an in-depth look at the clinical aspects of herbal treatment.

Online databases such as PubMed and the Cochrane Library are invaluable for accessing research studies and clinical trials on herbal remedies. Websites like the American Botanical Council and the National Center for Complementary and Integrative Health provide up-to-date information, safety guidelines, and efficacy reports on various herbs and supplements.

Local libraries and bookstores often carry a range of books on herbal medicine, from beginner's guides to comprehensive materia medica. Joining herbalist associations or local herb societies can connect you with experienced practitioners, workshops, and seminars that further your understanding and practical knowledge of herbal remedies.

Remember, while the internet offers a vast array of information, it's crucial to critically evaluate sources for credibility and reliability. Opt for information from well-respected authors, institutions, and peer-reviewed journals to ensure the accuracy and safety of the herbal practices you choose to incorporate into your life.

By weaving together insights from both historical texts and contemporary research, you can build a solid foundation for your practice of herbal medicine. Embrace the journey of learning, and let the wisdom of the ages guide you to a deeper connection with the natural world and your own well-being.

Further Reading and Study

Embarking on a deeper exploration of herbal remedies and natural healing, numerous resources can significantly enhance your understanding and practical skills. For those who have ignited a passion for herbalism through this book, expanding your knowledge through further reading and study is a natural next step. Engaging with a range of materials will broaden your perspective, offering insights into both the ancient traditions and the latest scientific research in herbal medicine. Consider delving into specialized books that focus on specific aspects of herbalism, such as ethnobotany, which examines the relationship between people and plants across different cultures. Texts on phytochemistry will unravel the complex chemical compounds in plants and their effects on human health. For a hands-on approach, practical guides on herbal gardening and wildcrafting provide invaluable knowledge on growing your own medicinal plants and ethically harvesting from the wild.

Subscribing to journals and magazines dedicated to herbal medicine is another excellent way to stay informed about the latest developments in the field. These publications often feature case studies, research findings, and interviews with experienced herbalists, enriching your learning with diverse perspectives.

Attending workshops, courses, and seminars offers a dynamic learning environment where you can gain practical experience and direct mentorship from seasoned practitioners. Many communities have herbalism schools or local herbalists offering classes that cover a wide range of topics, from basic herbology to advanced clinical herbal medicine.

Online platforms and forums dedicated to herbalism serve as vibrant communities for sharing experiences, asking questions, and connecting with fellow herbal enthusiasts. Engaging in these online spaces can provide support and encouragement as you apply your knowledge and experiment with creating your own remedies.

By integrating these resources into your journey, you create a comprehensive learning path that not only deepens your understanding of herbal medicine but also connects you with a global community of like-minded individuals passionate about natural healing. This continuous pursuit of knowledge empowers you to take control of your health and well-being, guided by the wisdom of herbal traditions and the principles of holistic healing.

Herbal Suppliers and Tools

Finding the right herbal suppliers and tools is crucial for anyone embarking on the journey of creating their own herbal remedies. The quality of herbs and the tools you use can significantly impact the effectiveness and safety of your homemade products. When sourcing herbs, look for suppliers who prioritize organic, ethically harvested, and sustainably sourced materials. Organic herbs are free from pesticides and other chemicals, ensuring that your remedies are as pure and effective as possible. Ethically harvested herbs ensure that plant populations are preserved for future generations, while sustainably sourced herbs support the health of the environment.

For those just starting, local health food stores often carry a selection of high-quality dried herbs. However, for more variety and bulk options, online herbal suppliers can be invaluable. Look for suppliers with transparent sourcing practices and positive customer reviews. Some reputable online sources include Mountain Rose Herbs, Starwest Botanicals, and Frontier Co-op.

In addition to herbs, having the right tools is essential for preparing your remedies. Basic tools include:

- Mortar and pestle for grinding herbs
- Glass jars and bottles for storing tinctures, oils, and dried herbs
- Cheesecloth or a fine mesh strainer for filtering tinctures and infusions
- A digital scale for precise measurements
- Labels and a waterproof marker for labeling your creations

Safety is paramount when preparing and using herbal remedies. Always use clean tools to prevent contamination and clearly label your remedies with the ingredients, date of creation, and suggested use. Start with small batches to test for personal sensitivities and effectiveness before making larger quantities.

By choosing high-quality herbs and utilizing the proper tools, you can ensure that your homemade herbal remedies are safe, effective, and tailored to your health needs. Remember, the journey to natural health is not only about the destination but also about understanding and enjoying the process of creating and using your own herbal products.

Glossary and Index

The Glossary and Index section serves as a comprehensive resource to enhance understanding and navigation of "The Lost Bible of Herbal Remedies." This segment is meticulously organized to provide quick access to detailed descriptions, ensuring readers can efficiently locate information on herbal remedies, preparation techniques, and health conditions addressed throughout the book.

Glossary: A curated list of terms and phrases commonly used in herbal medicine, each accompanied by a concise definition. This includes botanical terms, preparation methods (e.g., tincture, infusion, decoction), and common ailments. The glossary is designed to demystify technical language, making the rich world of herbal remedies accessible to beginners. For instance, "Adaptogen" is defined as a natural substance considered to help the body adapt to stress and to exert a normalizing effect upon bodily processes.

Index: An alphabetically arranged list of subjects, herbs, health conditions, and remedies covered in the book. Each entry in the index points to the page number where the topic is discussed, facilitating easy reference. Whether readers are looking for specific information on an herb like Echinacea, a remedy for a common ailment such as indigestion, or a general concept like "harvesting techniques," the index provides a straightforward pathway to the relevant content.

This dual structure supports readers in quickly finding the information they need, enhancing their learning experience, and applying the book's insights to their personal health and wellness journeys. By offering clear, accessible definitions and a user-friendly guide to the book's contents, the Glossary and Index empower readers to deepen their understanding of herbal medicine, engage more confidently with the material, and apply their knowledge to improve their health and well-being naturally.

Appendices

The Appendices serve as a practical toolkit, enhancing your herbal journey with essential resources. This section is meticulously designed to provide immediate access to a wealth of supplementary materials, ensuring you have everything you need to confidently embark on your path to natural healing.

Plant Index: A comprehensive list of all plants mentioned throughout the book, organized alphabetically. This index is your quick reference to the botanical world explored in our pages, offering insights into each plant's healing properties and uses.

Condition Index: Tailored to offer swift guidance, this index lists common ailments and directs you to herbal remedies discussed in the book. Whether you're seeking relief from a headache or looking for digestive support, this index simplifies your search for natural solutions.

Herbal Suppliers and Tools: Identifying trusted sources for high-quality herbs and the right tools for your herbal practice can be daunting. This section provides a curated list of reputable suppliers and essential tools, ensuring you have access to the best resources for crafting your remedies.

Glossary: Herbalism comes with its own language. The glossary demystifies terms and phrases, from "adaptogen" to "tincture," making the science of herbal medicine accessible to all, regardless of your background or experience level.

Further Reading and Study: Expanding your knowledge is a continuous journey. This curated selection of books, websites, and journals offers avenues for deeper exploration into the art and science of herbal remedies, encouraging lifelong learning and discovery.

By providing these resources, the Appendices aim to support your ongoing exploration and application of herbal medicine. With this toolkit at your disposal, you're well-equipped to navigate the world of natural healing, crafting remedies that nurture health and well-being for yourself and your loved ones.

Plant Index

The Plant Index serves as a vital tool for anyone delving into the world of herbal remedies, offering a gateway to understanding the myriad of plants discussed throughout this guide. Each entry within this index is meticulously organized to provide not only the common name of the plant but also its botanical counterpart, ensuring clarity and aiding in the accurate identification of each species. This section is designed to be an accessible reference, enabling readers to quickly locate information on the specific healing properties, traditional uses, and preparation methods for a wide range of medicinal plants.

- Starting with **Aloe Vera,** known botanically as **Aloe barbadensis miller**, this plant is renowned for its soothing, healing properties, particularly in the treatment of skin conditions and burns. It also plays a role in digestive health, offering relief from constipation and supporting overall gut health.

- Moving to **Arnica montana**, this herb is celebrated for its potent anti-inflammatory properties, making it a go-to remedy for bruises, sprains, and muscle soreness. Its application in the form of creams, salves, and tinctures highlights the versatility of herbal remedies in addressing physical discomfort.

- **Burdock Root**, or **Arctium lappa**, is another pivotal entry, known for its blood purifying and detoxifying effects. It has a long-standing history in herbal medicine for treating skin disorders such as eczema and psoriasis, showcasing the deep-rooted connection between internal health and external wellbeing.

- **Calendula officinalis**, commonly referred to as Calendula, offers remarkable healing abilities, particularly in wound healing and reducing inflammation. Its gentle nature makes it suitable for a wide range of topical applications, including cuts, scrapes, and even as an ingredient in natural beauty products.

- **Dandelion**, with its botanical name **Taraxacum officinale**, is often underestimated for its medicinal benefits. Beyond its common appearance in lawns and gardens, Dandelion is a powerhouse of nutrition, supporting liver health, digestion, and serving as a natural diuretic.

- **Echinacea**, known scientifically as **Echinacea purpurea**, stands out for its immune-boosting capabilities. Its use in preventing and treating the common cold and other respiratory infections underscores the critical role of natural remedies in supporting the body's defense mechanisms.

Each of these plants represents just the beginning of the vast botanical world explored in this guide. The Plant Index continues to unfold, offering insights into more plants with unique healing properties and applications. From Ginger, Zingiber officinale, known for its anti-inflammatory and digestive health benefits, to Lavender, Lavandula angustifolia, celebrated for its calming and soothing effects, the diversity of plants and their potential to enhance health and wellbeing is boundless.

As we progress through the index, the focus on easily accessible, safe, and effective herbal solutions remains paramount. This approach ensures that readers, regardless of their prior knowledge or experience with herbal medicine, can confidently explore and utilize the natural healing powers of plants. The journey through the Plant Index is designed to be both educational and empowering, providing a solid foundation for integrating herbal remedies into one's daily life for improved health and wellness.

- **Lemon Balm**, or **Melissa officinalis**, is cherished for its ability to ease stress and anxiety, improve sleep, and support digestive health. Its gentle lemon scent and flavor make it a popular choice for calming teas and aromatherapy blends. This herb's versatility extends to topical applications, where it is used to treat cold sores and other skin irritations due to its antiviral properties.

- **Nettle**, scientifically known as **Urtica dioica**, is a nutrient-rich plant that has been used for centuries to treat a variety of conditions including allergies, anemia, and arthritis. Its leaves are packed with vitamins and minerals, making it an excellent tonic for boosting overall health and vitality. Nettle is also known for its ability to support the body's detoxification processes and improve urinary tract health.

- **Oregano**, or **Origanum vulgare**, is widely recognized not just as a culinary herb but also for its powerful antibacterial and antioxidant properties. It is commonly used in oil form to treat respiratory conditions, digestive problems, and to boost the immune system. Oregano's active compounds, such as carvacrol and thymol, contribute to its therapeutic effects.

- **Peppermint, Mentha piperita**, is another herb that bridges the gap between culinary and medicinal uses. Its cooling effect is beneficial for relieving nausea, headaches, and digestive issues. Peppermint oil is particularly effective for irritable bowel syndrome (IBS) and has been widely studied for its ability to relax the gastrointestinal tract.

- **Rosemary**, Rosmarinus officinalis, is not only cherished for its aromatic qualities in cooking but also for its cognitive and circulatory benefits. It has been traditionally used to improve memory, alleviate muscle pain, and stimulate hair growth. Rosemary's rich antioxidant content also makes it a natural preservative with antimicrobial properties.

- **Sage, Salvia officinalis**, has a long history of use for its digestive, cognitive, and anti-inflammatory effects. It is particularly beneficial for sore throats, dental abscesses, and gingivitis when used as a mouthwash. Sage also has estrogenic properties, making it a helpful herb for managing symptoms of menopause.

- **Thyme, Thymus vulgaris**, is valued for its antiseptic and antifungal properties, making it an effective remedy for respiratory infections, coughs, and bronchitis. Its active compound, thymol, is used in many over-the-counter cough syrups and mouthwashes for its therapeutic effects.

- **Valerian, Valeriana officinalis**, is best known for its sedative qualities, making it a popular choice for treating insomnia and anxiety. Its root contains compounds that help to calm the nervous system and promote relaxation, offering a natural alternative to pharmaceutical sleep aids.

- **Yarrow, Achillea millefolium**, is a versatile herb known for its ability to stop bleeding, heal wounds, and reduce inflammation. It has been used traditionally in battlefield medicine and is also effective in treating digestive issues and promoting skin health.

- **Zinc** is not an herb but a mineral that's crucial for immune function, wound healing, and DNA synthesis. While not directly related to herbal remedies, its inclusion highlights the importance of a holistic approach to health, emphasizing the role of nutrients in conjunction with herbal treatments for optimal wellness.

This comprehensive exploration of medicinal plants and their benefits underscores the incredible diversity and potential of the natural world for supporting health and healing. From the soothing properties of Lemon Balm to the nutrient-rich offerings of Nettle, each plant holds a unique place in the herbal medicine cabinet. By understanding and harnessing these natural remedies, individuals can take proactive steps towards enhancing their health and well-being in harmony with nature.

Comprehensive List of Plants Mentioned

- **Aloe Vera**, scientifically known as **Aloe barbadensis miller**, is celebrated for its extensive use in skincare and digestive health. Its gel is a common remedy for burns, including sunburns, and its juice is used to aid digestion and alleviate constipation. This versatility makes Aloe Vera a staple in many households.

- **Arnica montana**, known for its anti-inflammatory properties, is often applied topically to reduce bruising and swelling associated with injuries. Its effectiveness in pain relief, especially for osteoarthritis, is supported by its use in various creams and ointments.

- **Burdock Root**, or **Arctium lappa**, plays a significant role in traditional herbal medicine as a blood purifier and a treatment for skin conditions like eczema and psoriasis. Its inclusion in teas and supplements underscores its detoxifying properties.

- **Calendula officinalis**, commonly referred to as Calendula, is utilized for its wound-healing and anti-inflammatory benefits. It is a gentle herb, often found in creams and salves for cuts, wounds, and other skin irritations, promoting rapid healing.

- **Dandelion, Taraxacum officinale**, is more than just a common weed; it's a powerhouse of nutrition that supports liver function, digestion, and serves as a natural diuretic. Both its leaves and roots are used in herbal remedies, showcasing the plant's versatility.

- **Echinacea**, or **Echinacea purpurea**, is widely recognized for its immune-boosting capabilities. It is commonly used at the onset of colds and flu to enhance the body's immune response, available in various forms including teas, capsules, and tinctures.

- **Ginger, Zingiber officinale**, is a well-known digestive aid and anti-inflammatory herb. It's used in numerous forms, from fresh or dried in cooking to powdered in supplements, addressing issues from nausea and indigestion to inflammatory conditions.

- **Lavender, Lavandula angustifolia**, is prized for its calming and soothing properties. Its essential oil is used in aromatherapy to reduce stress and improve sleep quality, while the dried flowers may be used in teas or baths for relaxation.

- **Milk Thistle, Silybum marianum**, is recognized for its liver-protective qualities. It is often used to support liver health, detoxify the body, and promote skin health, reflecting the interconnectedness of internal and external well-being.

- **Peppermint, Mentha piperita**, offers relief from digestive discomforts such as irritable bowel syndrome (IBS) and nausea. Its cooling effect is also beneficial in topical applications for headaches and muscle pain.

- **Rosemary, Rosmarinus officinalis**, not only enhances culinary dishes but also boosts memory, improves circulation, and relieves muscle pain when used in herbal preparations. Its antioxidant properties further support its use in natural beauty products.

- **Sage, Salvia officinalis**, with its antiseptic and anti-inflammatory benefits, is commonly used in gargles and mouthwashes to soothe sore throats and treat dental abscesses. It also has applications in menopausal symptom relief due to its estrogenic effects.

- **Thyme, Thymus vulgaris**, is valued for its antibacterial and cough-relieving properties. It is a key ingredient in natural cough remedies and has a long history of use in respiratory health.

- **Valerian, Valeriana officinalis**, is best known for its sedative and anxiety-reducing effects. It is often used in herbal formulations to improve sleep quality and manage stress, showcasing the plant's adaptogenic properties.

- **Yarrow, Achillea millefolium**, is recognized for its ability to stop bleeding and heal wounds. Its broad application in herbal first aid kits, along with its use in digestive and reproductive health, underscores its versatility in natural medicine.

These plants represent just a portion of the vast botanical knowledge contained within the realm of herbal remedies. Each offers unique benefits and applications, contributing to a holistic approach to health and wellness that harnesses the power of nature.

- **Hawthorn, Crataegus monogyna**, stands out for its cardiovascular benefits, particularly in enhancing heart health and circulation. Traditionally used to treat heart failure, high blood pressure, and digestive issues, Hawthorn is a testament to the heart's symbolic and physical significance in herbal medicine. Its berries, leaves, and flowers are utilized in various preparations, showcasing its versatility.

- **St. John's Wort, Hypericum perforatum**, is renowned for its antidepressant and anti-inflammatory properties. It's commonly used for treating mild to moderate depression, anxiety, and wounds. Care should be taken, as it interacts with several medications, highlighting the importance of knowledgeable guidance in herbal remedy use.

- **Turmeric, Curcuma longa**, has gained popularity for its potent anti-inflammatory and antioxidant effects. Its active compound, curcumin, contributes to its efficacy in treating arthritis, heart disease, and various other conditions. Turmeric is often used in powder form, adding both color and health benefits to dishes.

- **Slippery Elm, Ulmus rubra**, is valued for its soothing properties, particularly in the digestive system. It forms a gel-like substance when mixed with water, providing relief for throat irritation, coughs, and gastrointestinal issues. Its bark is the primary part used, demonstrating the diverse sources of healing within plants.

- **Licorice Root, Glycyrrhiza glabra**, is known for its sweet flavor and extensive medicinal properties, including soothing gastrointestinal problems, treating respiratory issues, and supporting adrenal function. However, its use is cautioned due to potential effects on blood pressure and potassium levels, underscoring the need for balance and expertise in herbal applications.

- **Elderberry, Sambucus nigra**, has been used for centuries to boost the immune system and combat colds and flu. Its berries and flowers are packed with antioxidants and vitamins, making it a popular choice for natural immune support in various forms, including syrups, teas, and supplements.

- **Lemon Balm, Melissa officinalis**, is cherished for its ability to ease stress and anxiety, improve sleep, and support digestive health. Its gentle lemon scent and flavor make it a popular choice for calming teas and aromatherapy blends. This herb's versatility extends to topical applications, where it is used to treat cold sores and other skin irritations due to its antiviral properties.

- **Nettle, Urtica dioica**, is a nutrient-rich plant that has been used for centuries to treat a variety of conditions including allergies, anemia, and arthritis. Its leaves are packed with vitamins and minerals, making it an excellent tonic for boosting overall health and vitality. Nettle is also known for its ability to support the body's detoxification processes and improve urinary tract health.

- **Oregano, Origanum vulgare**, is widely recognized not just as a culinary herb but also for its powerful antibacterial and antioxidant properties. It is commonly used in oil form to treat respiratory conditions, digestive problems, and to boost the immune system. Oregano's active compounds, such as carvacrol and thymol, contribute to its therapeutic effects.

- **Plantain, Plantago major**, is often overlooked as a common weed, yet it possesses powerful medicinal properties, particularly for skin health and wound healing. Its leaves can be applied topically to soothe insect bites, cuts, and burns, or used internally to aid digestion and respiratory health.

- **Goldenseal, Hydrastis canadensis**, is revered for its antimicrobial and anti-inflammatory properties. It's commonly used to treat digestive and respiratory infections, showcasing the importance of natural antibiotics in herbal medicine. Due to its overharvesting, responsible sourcing of Goldenseal is crucial.

- **Chamomile, Matricaria chamomilla**, is widely known for its calming effects, making it a go-to remedy for stress, anxiety, and sleep issues. Its gentle nature makes it suitable for all ages, often found in teas and topical applications for its soothing properties on the skin and digestive system.

- **Ginkgo Biloba**, known for its cognitive-enhancing properties, has been used in traditional medicine to improve memory, concentration, and blood circulation. Its leaves are utilized in extracts and supplements, representing the integration of ancient plants into modern health practices.

By exploring the vast array of plants mentioned in this guide, readers are equipped with the knowledge to harness the healing power of nature. Each plant offers a unique contribution to health and wellness, emphasizing the importance of diversity and personalization in herbal medicine. With this comprehensive understanding, individuals can confidently incorporate herbal remedies into their journey towards natural health and healing.

Condition Index

The Condition Index serves as an essential tool for anyone venturing into the world of herbal remedies, providing a comprehensive guide to addressing a wide array of health concerns with natural solutions. This index is meticulously organized to help you quickly identify which herbs may be beneficial for specific conditions, from common ailments like colds and flu to more chronic issues such as arthritis and digestive disorders. Each entry in the index is accompanied by a brief overview of the condition, followed by a list of herbs that have been traditionally used to alleviate symptoms or address the root cause of the problem.

For instance, if you're seeking natural ways to enhance digestive health, the index will direct you to herbs such as peppermint, known for its soothing properties on the gastrointestinal tract, or ginger, celebrated for its ability to relieve nausea and improve digestion. Similarly, those looking to support respiratory health might find recommendations for herbs like mullein, which has a long history of use in treating coughs and respiratory conditions, or elderberry, recognized for its immune-boosting capabilities that can help ward off colds and flu.

The Condition Index also highlights the importance of understanding each herb's properties and how they interact with the body, emphasizing the need for a holistic approach to health. It's not just about treating symptoms but nurturing overall well-being by choosing herbs that align with your body's needs and natural rhythms. Moreover, the index provides guidance on how to use these herbs effectively, whether as teas, tinctures, capsules, or topical applications, ensuring you have the knowledge to prepare remedies safely and with confidence.

Safety is a paramount concern when using herbal remedies, and the Condition Index addresses this by noting any potential side effects or interactions with medications for each herb listed. This information empowers you to make informed decisions about incorporating herbs into your health regimen, particularly if you are managing chronic conditions or taking prescription drugs.

As you explore the Condition Index, you'll discover the versatility of herbal medicine and its potential to support health in a variety of ways. Whether you're a beginner to herbal remedies or looking to expand your knowledge, this index is designed to be an invaluable resource on your journey to natural health and wellness. By providing a bridge between traditional wisdom and modern science, it encourages a balanced and informed approach to healing, reminding us of the profound connection between the plant world and our own well-being.

Expanding upon the foundation laid for understanding the therapeutic applications of herbs, the Condition Index delves deeper into addressing specific health concerns with targeted herbal remedies. For those grappling with stress and anxiety, adaptogenic herbs such as ashwagandha and holy basil offer a natural means to restore balance and resilience to the body's stress response systems. These herbs have been revered for centuries in traditional medicine for their ability to enhance mental clarity and promote a sense of calm.

In the realm of skin care, the healing properties of calendula and tea tree oil emerge as potent allies. Calendula, with its anti-inflammatory and antimicrobial qualities, is excellent for soothing and healing irritated skin, making it an ideal choice for treating eczema and psoriasis. Tea tree oil, known for its antiseptic properties, provides a natural solution for acne and other bacterial skin infections, underscoring the versatility of herbal remedies in addressing a range of dermatological issues.

For individuals seeking relief from joint pain and inflammation, the anti-arthritic properties of herbs like turmeric and ginger come to the forefront. These herbs contain compounds that have been scientifically proven to reduce inflammation and alleviate pain, offering a complementary approach to managing conditions such as arthritis and fibromyalgia. By incorporating these herbs into one's daily regimen, either through dietary intake or topical application, one can harness their analgesic and anti-inflammatory benefits.

The Condition Index also sheds light on the role of herbs in supporting cardiovascular health. Hawthorn, for instance, stands out for its ability to strengthen the heart and improve circulation, making it a valuable herb for those dealing with high blood pressure or congestive heart failure. Similarly, garlic's ability to lower cholesterol levels and improve arterial health highlights the potential of herbal remedies in preventing heart disease and enhancing overall cardiovascular function.

Furthermore, the index explores the use of herbs in boosting cognitive function and memory. Ginkgo biloba, with its ability to enhance blood flow to the brain, offers promise for improving cognitive performance and slowing the progression of age-related cognitive decline. Lion's mane mushroom, another cognitive enhancer, supports nerve growth and brain health, illustrating the growing interest in nootropic herbs for mental wellness.

Digestive health is another area where herbal remedies can make a significant impact. Peppermint and ginger, for instance, are not only effective in relieving nausea and indigestion but also promote healthy digestion and soothe gastrointestinal discomfort. These herbs, along with others like fennel and chamomile, demonstrate the holistic approach of herbal medicine in treating the body as an interconnected system, where improving one aspect of health can benefit the whole.

In addressing women's health issues, herbs such as red raspberry leaf and chasteberry offer natural support for menstrual and hormonal imbalances, providing relief from symptoms associated with PMS and menopause. These herbs, celebrated for their gentle yet effective action, underscore the potential of plant-based remedies in fostering female reproductive health and well-being.

The Condition Index, in its comprehensive exploration of herbal remedies, not only guides individuals in selecting the right herbs for their specific health concerns but also emphasizes the importance of integrating these natural solutions into a balanced lifestyle. By doing so, it encourages a proactive approach to health, where prevention and self-care go hand in hand with the healing power of nature. Through this holistic perspective, the index serves as a testament to the enduring wisdom of herbal medicine and its relevance in today's health-conscious society.

Quick Reference for Ailments and Remedies

Quick Reference for Ailments and Remedies serves as a practical guide for those seeking to address health concerns with natural, herbal solutions. This section is designed to provide immediate, accessible information on using herbs to treat a variety of common conditions, emphasizing the importance of integrating these natural remedies into a holistic health strategy.

For digestive issues such as indigestion, bloating, and nausea, herbs like ginger, peppermint, and chamomile are invaluable.

- Ginger, with its potent anti-inflammatory properties, can be used to make a simple tea that soothes the stomach and aids digestion.
- Peppermint, known for its ability to relax the gastrointestinal tract, can be taken as a tea or in capsule form to alleviate symptoms of IBS and other digestive discomforts.
- Chamomile, often celebrated for its calming effects, also serves as a gentle remedy for upset stomachs, promoting relaxation and aiding in digestive health.

When it comes to respiratory health, herbs such as elderberry, echinacea, and thyme offer support, especially during cold and flu season.

- Elderberry syrup is a popular choice for its immune-boosting properties and can help reduce the duration and severity of cold symptoms.
- Echinacea, taken at the onset of a cold, can support the body's immune response, while thyme has been used traditionally in herbal teas and syrups to ease coughs and sore throats, thanks to its antiseptic and expectorant properties.

Skin and hair care concerns, including acne, eczema, and hair loss, can also be addressed with herbal remedies.

- Tea tree oil, with its powerful antibacterial and antifungal qualities, is effective in treating acne when diluted and applied to the skin.
- Aloe vera gel is renowned for its soothing and healing properties, making it an excellent treatment for eczema and other skin irritations.
- For hair loss, rosemary and lavender essential oils can be massaged into the scalp to stimulate hair growth and improve circulation.

Pain and inflammation, common issues that affect many, can be managed with herbs like turmeric, willow bark, and ginger.

- Turmeric, containing the active compound curcumin, is highly regarded for its anti-inflammatory and antioxidant effects, making it beneficial for conditions such as arthritis and other inflammatory disorders.
- Willow bark, often referred to as "nature's aspirin," has been used for centuries to relieve pain and reduce inflammation.
- Ginger, either consumed as a tea or applied topically as a compress, offers relief from muscle soreness and joint pain due to its anti-inflammatory properties.

Mental health and well-being, including stress, anxiety, and depression, can be positively influenced by herbs such as lavender, chamomile, and lemon balm.

- Lavender, used in aromatherapy or as a tea, is well-known for its ability to reduce stress and promote relaxation.
- Chamomile tea, with its mild sedative effects, can help alleviate anxiety and improve sleep quality.
- Lemon balm, either taken as a tea or in capsule form, has been shown to improve mood and cognitive function, offering a natural remedy for those dealing with stress and anxiety.

As we continue to explore the vast world of herbal remedies, it's important to remember that the effectiveness of these natural solutions can vary from person to person. Always consult with a healthcare professional before incorporating new herbal remedies into your regimen, especially if you are pregnant, nursing, or taking prescription medications.

Boosting the immune system is crucial, especially in times of increased stress and seasonal changes. Herbs like astragalus, garlic, and reishi mushrooms play a significant role in enhancing immune health.

- Astragalus, a staple in traditional Chinese medicine, is known for its ability to strengthen the body's defense against illness.
- Garlic, with its potent antiviral and antibacterial properties, can be easily incorporated into daily meals to support immune function.
- Reishi mushrooms, often referred to as the "mushroom of immortality," help to modulate the immune system, making the body more resilient to pathogens.

For those dealing with urinary tract infections (UTIs) and bladder issues, herbs such as cranberry, uva ursi, and dandelion offer natural relief.

- Cranberry prevents bacteria from adhering to the bladder walls, reducing the likelihood of infections.
- Uva ursi has antiseptic properties that aid in treating urinary tract infections, while dandelion acts as a diuretic, helping to flush out bacteria from the urinary system.

Cardiovascular health is another area where herbal remedies can make a significant impact.

- Hawthorn berry is renowned for its cardiovascular benefits, including improving heart function, preventing heart disease, and managing high blood pressure.
- Garlic also contributes to heart health by lowering cholesterol levels and improving circulation.

Digestive health can be supported with herbs like licorice root, peppermint, and ginger.

- Licorice root soothes gastrointestinal issues and can heal stomach ulcers.
- Peppermint relieves symptoms of IBS and promotes healthy digestion.
- Ginger, beyond its anti-inflammatory benefits, stimulates digestion and relieves nausea.

For those seeking natural solutions for hormonal balance and reproductive health, herbs such as vitex (chasteberry), maca root, and red clover are invaluable.

- Vitex helps to regulate menstrual cycles and alleviate symptoms of PMS, while maca root supports overall hormone balance and fertility.
- Red clover contains phytoestrogens that can ease menopausal symptoms and improve reproductive health.

Sleep disorders and insomnia can be addressed with calming herbs like valerian root, passionflower, and hops.

- Valerian root is a powerful sedative that encourages deep, restorative sleep.
- Passionflower reduces anxiety and improves sleep quality, and hops have been used for centuries to treat sleeplessness and restlessness.

Herbal remedies also offer support for liver health, with herbs like milk thistle, dandelion root, and turmeric.

- Milk thistle is widely recognized for its liver-protective effects, aiding in detoxification and liver regeneration.
- Dandelion root supports liver function and digestion, while turmeric reduces inflammation and protects against liver damage.

In managing chronic conditions such as diabetes, herbs like cinnamon, fenugreek, and bitter melon can be beneficial.

- Cinnamon helps to regulate blood sugar levels
- fenugreek improves glucose tolerance
- bitter melon acts as a natural insulin to help control diabetes.

It's essential to approach herbal remedies with knowledge and respect, recognizing that while they offer incredible health benefits, they must be used responsibly. Consulting with a healthcare professional before starting any new herbal regimen ensures safe and effective use, especially for those with existing health conditions or those taking prescription medications. Through mindful integration of these natural solutions, individuals can enhance their well-being and lead a more balanced, healthy life.

References and Bibliography

The foundation of "The Lost Bible of Herbal Remedies" is built upon a wealth of knowledge derived from a variety of sources, ensuring the information presented is both accurate and reliable. This section acknowledges the contributions of those sources, providing readers with a pathway to further their understanding of herbal remedies and natural medicine.

Key references include seminal texts in the field of herbal medicine, such as

- "The Complete Herbal Handbook for Farm and Stable" by Juliette de Bairacli Levy, which offers invaluable insights into traditional herbal practices.

- "Medical Herbalism: The Science and Practice of Herbal Medicine" by David Hoffmann provides a thorough exploration of the scientific principles behind herbal medicine, making it a crucial resource for understanding the how and why behind herbal remedies.

- Research and studies from peer-reviewed journals such as the Journal of Ethnopharmacology and Phytotherapy Research have been instrumental in validating the efficacy of various herbal treatments mentioned throughout the book. These journals offer a bridge between traditional knowledge and modern scientific validation, ensuring the remedies are both safe and effective.

- For those interested in the cultivation and harvesting of medicinal plants, "The Organic Medicinal Herb Farmer" by Jeff Carpenter and Melanie Carpenter offers practical advice and insights into growing herbs sustainably.

- Safety and ethical considerations are paramount in herbal medicine, with "Herbal Contraindications and Drug Interactions" by Francis Brinker providing essential information on potential interactions between herbal remedies and conventional medications, ensuring the safe use of herbs.

- This book also draws upon the rich tradition of herbal medicine across cultures, with texts such as "Healing with the Herbs of Life" by Lesley Tierra and "The Practice of Traditional Western Herbalism" by Matthew Wood offering perspectives on Western, Ayurvedic, and Chinese herbal traditions.

- For additional learning and exploration, the American Botanical Council and the National Center for Complementary and Integrative Health offer extensive online resources, including databases and articles on herbal medicine, further enriching the reader's journey into the world of natural healing.

Cited Sources and Further Reading

The enriching journey through "The Lost Bible of Herbal Remedies" is supported by a foundation of authoritative sources and further reading that deepens your understanding of herbal medicine. These resources were meticulously selected to ensure the information provided is both comprehensive and reliable, catering to the curiosity and growth of beginners in herbalism.

For those eager to explore beyond the pages of this guide, the following texts and resources are recommended.

- "The Herbal Medicine-Maker's Handbook: A Home Manual" by James Green offers an engaging dive into crafting your own herbal remedies, emphasizing the practical aspects of herbalism.

- "The Modern Herbal Dispensatory: A Medicine-Making Guide" by Thomas Easley and Steven Horne provides detailed instructions on creating herbal formulations, from tinctures to salves, making it an invaluable resource for hands-on learning.

- Additionally, "Adaptogens: Herbs for Strength, Stamina, and Stress Relief" by David Winston and Steven Maimes, explores the unique category of herbs known as adaptogens, which support the body's natural ability to handle stress. This book is particularly beneficial for understanding how to incorporate these powerful herbs into daily life for improved resilience and well-being.

- For those interested in the scientific underpinnings of herbal medicine, "Principles and Practice of Phytotherapy: Modern Herbal Medicine" by Kerry Bone and Simon Mills delves into the evidence-based approach to herbal healing, offering a bridge between traditional wisdom and modern science.

Online resources also offer a wealth of information, with websites like the American Herbalists Guild and the Herb Society of America providing articles, research papers, and educational materials that are constantly updated, ensuring you stay informed on the latest in herbal medicine.

By engaging with these recommended sources, you not only expand your knowledge but also join a community of like-minded individuals passionate about natural health. This journey of discovery does not end here; it's a lifelong path of learning, healing, and growing with the natural world.

Thank You for Choosing

THE LOST BIBLE OF HERBAL REMEDIES

Dear Reader,

Thank you for embarking on this journey with me through the pages of "The Lost Bible of Herbal Remedies": Unlock the Power of Plants for Better Health and Healing Your Body the Natural Way. Your commitment to exploring the wonders of natural healing and herbal remedies is truly inspiring.

As a token of my gratitude, I am excited to present you with an exclusive gift:

The All-Inclusive Herbal Recipe Collection

This bonus chapter is designed to enrich your understanding and practice of herbal medicine, providing you with an array of recipes that harness the power of nature for your health and well-being.

I hope these recipes become a valuable part of your health journey, helping you to achieve lasting well-being and vitality.

Once again, thank you for choosing this book and for your dedication to natural health. Wishing you all the best on your path to holistic wellness.

Warm regards,

Emily Everleaf

TO GET YOUR EXCLUSIVE BONUSES SCAN THE QR CODE

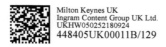

9 798332 663246